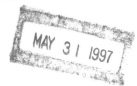
FIRST AID
── FOR ──
CHILDREN

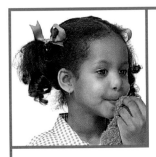
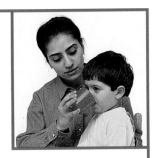
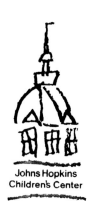

Johns Hopkins
Children's Center

FIRST AID
— FOR —
CHILDREN
FAST

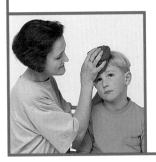
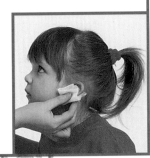

A DK PUBLISHING BOOK

Project Editor
Caroline Greene

Senior Art Editor
Jane Bull

US Editor
Jill Hamilton

Managing Art Editor
Tina Vaughan

Managing Editor
Jemima Dunne

DTP Designer
Karen Ruane

Production
Maryann Rogers

Photography
Andy Crawford and Steve Gorton

First American Edition, 1995
4 6 8 10 9 7 5
Published in the United States by
DK Publishing, Inc.
95 Madison Avenue,
New York, New York 10016

Library of Congress Cataloging-in-Publication Data

First aid for children fast. -- 1st American ed.
   p.   cm.
  Includes index.
  ISBN 1-56458-702-9
  1. Pediatric emergencies. 2. First aid in illness and injury.
RJ370.F58 1995
618.92'0025--dc20

94-26716
CIP

Reproduced in Italy by GRB Editrice, Verona
Printed and bound in the U.S.A. by R.R. Donnelley & Sons Co.

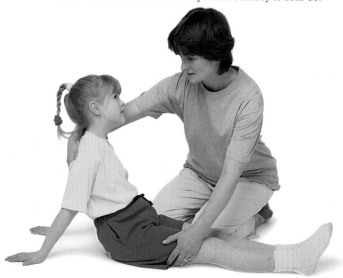

FOREWORD

As Maryland's regional pediatric shock trauma facility, the Johns Hopkins Children's Center is in the business of keeping children well. More than 30,000 infants, toddlers, and adolescents come to our emergency department each year, usually accompanied by frightened, frantic caregivers. That's why we hope you will take time to read this book *before* you need to use it, and share it with other caregivers.

It's also important to keep in mind that children aren't merely small adults. Their physical and emotional needs are unique. In emergency situations, they require assistance that is carefully tailored to their size and age. It's for those reasons that we also recommend you survey local hospitals. Which ones have equipment designed just for children? Do they have staffs trained to deal exclusively with kids? Those aren't things you want to leave to chance.

To learn more about the Johns Hopkins Children's Center approach to caring for children and their families, contact the Office of Public Affairs at 410-955-8662. Our Physician Referral Service is available weekdays at 1-800-45JOHNS.

We know you will find this book a partner in reaching the goal we share – the well-being of our children.

The Physicians and Staff
The Johns Hopkins Children's Center

CONTENTS

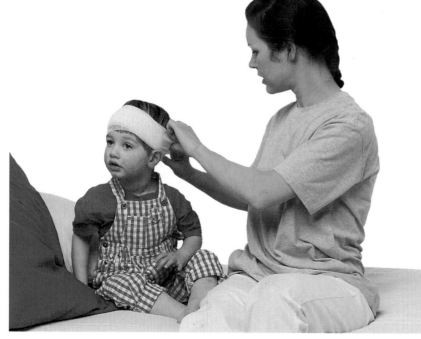

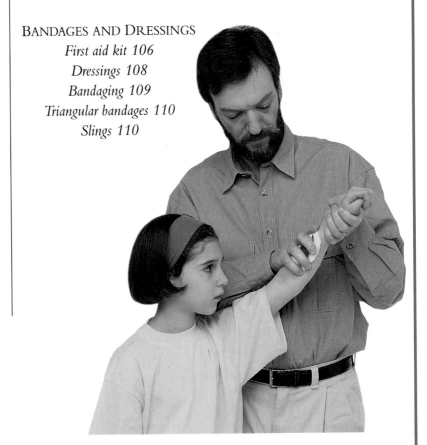

INTRODUCTION

This book has been compiled primarily for parents but also for others – grandparents, teachers, babysitters, playgroup leaders – who may regularly, or even occasionally, find themselves in charge of infants and children. The content has been set out in a clear and logical way and the information presented largely in pictorial form using simple words and captions to make it very easy to follow and to understand. The first aid methods and techniques described are in accordance with accepted modern practice and are in compliance with guidelines set out by the Emergency Cardiac Care Committee of the American Heart Association.

Emergencies are by their very nature unexpected events and require a prompt and proper response. If you follow the advice and guidance given in this book you will undoubtedly be able to give early and effective help whenever it is needed. You should be aware however that first aid is essentially a practical skill and your confidence and effectiveness will be greatly enhanced by expert training in a practical setting. The American Red Cross has chapters throughout the country and regularly runs a wide variety of first aid courses, some exclusively concerned with first aid for infants and children. You can find out more about these courses by telephoning your local Red Cross.

Giving first aid – coping with the emergency and doing the right thing promptly and effectively – can be straightforward but it can also be stressful, sometimes distasteful (especially if the child is not your own), and even dangerous. It is important that you remain in control of your feelings and avoid any tendency to an impulsive, rash action that could result in additional harm to an injured child or to yourself. You cannot give effective help if you yourself become a victim, so you must always take a little time to think before you act. This book is intended to help you to do the right thing at the right time – safely and effectively.

How to use this book

This book covers first aid treatment for everything from minor cuts to cardiopulmonary resuscitation. For every condition a series of photographs shows you exactly what to do in an emergency. Key pieces of information are indicated on the photographs and supplementary advice is given in the step-by-step text.

The injuries are organized by type, in sections such as Wounds and Bleeding or Bites and Stings. However, in an emergency, the thumbnail index on the back cover will direct you quickly to the relevant page.

There are also sections, such as Action in an Emergency and Bandages and Dressings, that contain information for general reference.

Key signs and symptoms help you recognize the conditions

Annotations highlight essential actions

Clear photographs illustrate every step of treatment

Symbols highlight the action necessary to access further medical attention

The quick reference index on the back cover gives instant access to major first aid emergencies

Cross-references direct you to information about related injuries

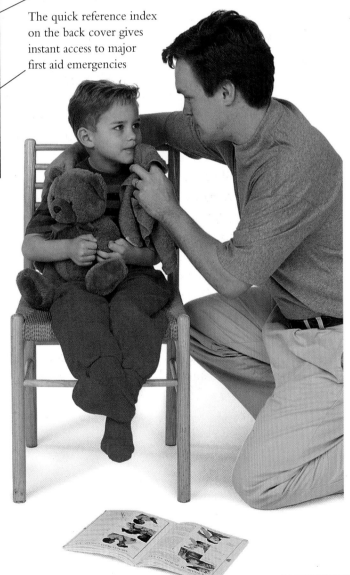

Guide to the symbols

The following appear if your child needs further medical attention:

ⓒ CALL A DOCTOR
(Telephone for further advice.)

✚ TAKE YOUR CHILD TO THE HOSPITAL
(Your child needs to be seen in the emergency room.)

☎ CALL 911 OR YOUR LOCAL EMS
(Your child needs urgent medical attention and is best transported by ambulance to the hospital.)

☠ CALL YOUR POISON CONTROL CENTER
(Call for advice concerning poisons.)

9

ACTION IN AN EMERGENCY

**In any emergency, particularly one involving children,
it is important to keep calm and act logically. Remember these four steps:**

1 Assess the situation

- What happened?
- How did it happen?
- Is there more than one injured child?
- Is there any continuing danger?
- Is there anyone who can help?
- Do I need an ambulance?

2 Think of safety

- Do not risk injuring yourself – you cannot help if you become a victim.
- Remove any source of danger from your child or move your child to safety.
- Move your child only if you must, and do so very carefully to prevent further injury.

3 Treat serious injuries first

In children, there are two conditions that immediately threaten life:

- *Inability to breathe* (see ABC OF RESUSCITATION, p.14)
- *Serious bleeding* (see BLEEDING, p.46).

If more than one child is injured go to the quiet one first – he may be unconscious.

10

4 Get help

Shout for help early to bring others to your assistance – ask them to • Call a doctor or an ambulance • Move a child to safety, if necessary • Make the area safe • Help with first aid.

Telephoning for help

When you call 911 or your local EMS, ask for an ambulance and give the following information:

- Your telephone number
- The accident location
- The type of accident
- The number, sex, and age of the victims
- Details about their condition
- Details of any hazards, such as spilled gasoline.

Always let the dispatcher hang up first.

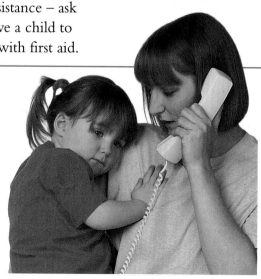

FIRE

Have an escape plan

Before an emergency happens, decide:
- *How would you get out of each room?*
- *How do you help babies and small children?*
- *Where will you meet when you've escaped?*

SKILLET FIRE • *Turn off stove* • *Cover pan with lid, wet dish towel, or fire blanket – leave this on for half an hour* • *DO NOT throw water over the flames* • *If not under control, close the door, call the fire department, get everyone out of the house.*

Escaping from a fire

1 Feel the door. If the door is cool, leave the room. If it is hot, see step 2.

REMEMBER • *Carry out babies and toddlers* • *Children over six should look after only themselves when escaping – don't ask them to do anything else*
- *Close all doors behind you*
- *Meet outside your house*
- *NEVER go back inside* • *Phone for help from somewhere else.*

2 If the door is hot, don't open it. Go to the window.

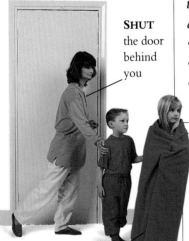

SHUT the door behind you

LEAVE quickly
DO NOT GO BACK

IF *you have to escape through the window, slide your child out, hang onto him, then tell him to drop to the ground. Slide out yourself, hang from the ledge, then drop. If you have to break the glass first, put a blanket over the frame before escaping.*

PLACE blanket to keep smoke out

KEEP children low, where air is clearest

OPEN window, call for help; hang towel to attract attention

Clothing on fire

If no water is available

Wrap the child tightly in a coat or blanket (not synthetic), or other heavy fabric. Lay him down and roll him to stifle the flames.

If water is available

Lay the child down with the burning side uppermost and douse the child with water.

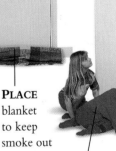

DO NOT *let the child run about in a panic; rapid movement will fan the flames.*

IF *your own clothes catch fire, wrap yourself up in heavy material, lie down, and roll.*

11

ELECTRICAL INJURY

If an electrical current passes through a child's body, it may cause breathing and even the heart to stop. The current may cause burns both where it enters and leaves the body. Alternating current (AC) causes muscle spasms that can prevent a child from letting go of an electric cord.

CONTACT *with high-voltage current, found in power lines and overhead cables, is usually fatal for a child. Severe burns result and the child may be thrown some distance from the point of contact.* **NEVER** *approach the injured child unless you are told officially that the power has been cut off, or you will be in danger from "arcing," or "jumping," high-voltage electricity.*

Low-voltage current

Children are at risk of suffering an electric shock if they play with electrical sockets or plugs, or if they bring an electrical appliance into contact with water.

IF *the child seems unharmed, make him rest and observe his condition.* ✆ CALL A DOCTOR

1 Break the contact by switching off the current at the circuit breaker.

2 If you cannot switch off the current, stand on dry insulating material such as telephone books, or a wooden box. Use a wooden broom handle or chair to push the child's limbs away from the source.

IF *the child loses consciousness, assess his condition (see* UNCONSCIOUS BABY, *p.16;* UNCONSCIOUS CHILD, *p.22). Be prepared to resuscitate. If he is breathing, place him in the* RECOVERY POSITION *(see p.24).*

DO NOT *touch the child's skin with your hands. Pull at his clothes only as a last resort.*

STAND on insulating material

PUSH the source away

3 Without touching the child, wrap a dry towel around his feet and pull him away from the source.

☎ CALL 911 OR YOUR LOCAL EMS

WRAP a dry towel around his feet. Pull him away

DROWNING

Babies and young children can drown quickly if they slip into a pool or pond or are left unattended in a bath. Even 1in (2.5cm) of water is enough to cover a baby's nose and mouth if she falls forward.

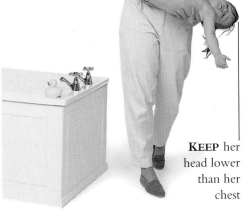

A CHILD may get into difficulty in open water, especially if it is turbulent or very cold. Rescue him quickly. Try to reach him from the shore or bank with your hand or a stick, or throw him a rope. Get him dry and warm as quickly as possible (see also HYPOTHERMIA, p.94).

1 Lift your child out of the water. Carry her with her head lower than her chest.

2 ☎ CALL 911 OR YOUR LOCAL EMS OR ✚ TAKE HER TO THE HOSPITAL, even if she seems recovered, since she may have inhaled water, causing lung damage.

KEEP her head lower than her chest

The unconscious child

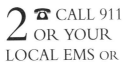

CHECK his pulse

OPEN airway

CHECK for breathing

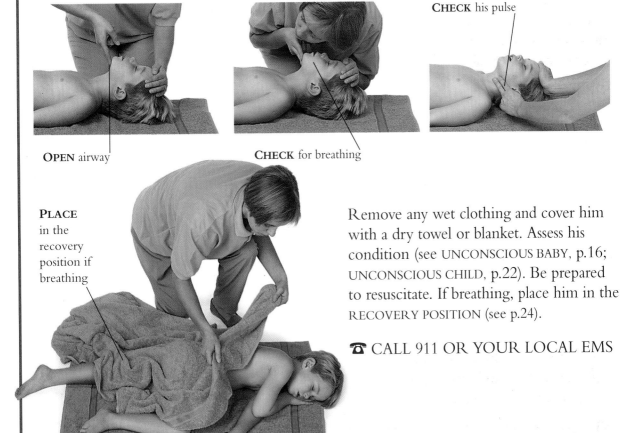

PLACE in the recovery position if breathing

Remove any wet clothing and cover him with a dry towel or blanket. Assess his condition (see UNCONSCIOUS BABY, p.16; UNCONSCIOUS CHILD, p.22). Be prepared to resuscitate. If breathing, place him in the RECOVERY POSITION (see p.24).

☎ CALL 911 OR YOUR LOCAL EMS

13

ABC OF RESUSCITATION

A baby or child who stops breathing will become unconscious because no oxygen reaches the brain. Lack of oxygen also causes the heartbeat to slow down until it stops altogether. If your child is unconscious and stops breathing, you need to clear your child's airway and breathe into the lungs (Artificial Respiration). If the heartbeat has stopped, you need to force blood to your child's brain with chest compressions. This combination of Artificial Respiration and chest compressions is Cardiopulmonary Resuscitation (CPR).

FOR *a-step-by-step guide to* RESUSCITATING A BABY *see p. 16.* **FOR** *a step-by-step guide to* RESUSCITATING A CHILD *see p. 22.*

ASSESS your baby and act on your findings

ASSESS your child and act on your findings

14

A is for airway

You need to open the air passage, or airway. Look for and remove any obstruction in the mouth. Tilt the head and lift the chin to bring the tongue away from the back of the throat. Do not tilt the head if you suspect a neck injury.

For a baby

For a child

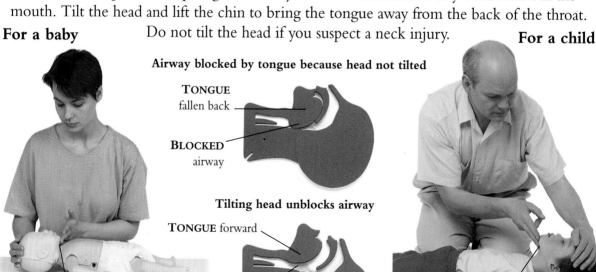

Airway blocked by tongue because head not tilted

TONGUE fallen back

BLOCKED airway

Tilting head unblocks airway

TONGUE forward

UNBLOCKED airway

TILT the head only slightly

TILT the head back to open the airway

B is for breathing

For a baby

If your child is not breathing after the airway is opened, you can blow your exhaled air into the lungs to get oxygen into the child's blood.

For a child

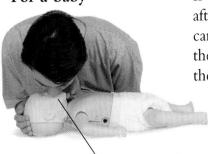

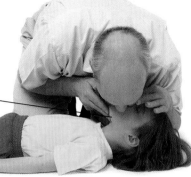

HOLD the nose and blow into the mouth

BREATHE gently into the mouth and nose until the chest rises

C is for circulation

For a baby

If your baby's or child's heart has stopped and there is no pulse, giving chest compressions will drive blood through the heart and around the body. This is always combined with Artificial Respiration. The combination of techniques is known as CPR – Cardiopulmonary Resuscitation.

For a child

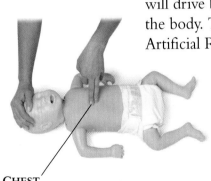

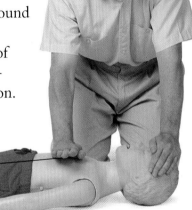

CHEST COMPRESSIONS are given with one hand only

CHEST COMPRESSIONS are given with two fingers

Assessing the situation

For a baby you need to determine three things:

1 Is the baby conscious?

2 Is the baby breathing?

3 Is there a pulse?

Before you rush to help a baby or child, you must decide whether there is any continuing danger (such as fire, fumes, or electricity) to the child or to yourself. You cannot assist if you become a victim. Shout for help if there is someone within earshot. Always try to remove the danger from the child, and move an injured child only if you must.

For a child you need to determine three things:

1 Is the child conscious?

2 Is the child breathing?

3 Is there a pulse?

UNCONSCIOUS BABY

Assess your baby's condition.

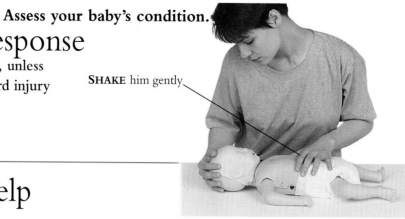

1 Check for response

- Shake your baby gently, unless you suspect a spinal cord injury
- Call his name
- Pinch his skin

SHAKE him gently

2 Shout for help

3 Open the airway

- Remove any obvious obstruction from mouth
- Use one finger to lift the chin
- Tilt the head back very slightly

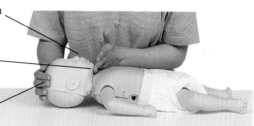

LOOK in mouth

LIFT chin with one finger

TILT head back very slightly

4 Check for breathing

- Listen for sounds of breathing
- Feel for breath on your cheek
- Look along the chest for movement
- Check for at least five seconds before deciding whether the baby is breathing

LISTEN for breathing

LOOK for chest movements

FEEL for breath on your cheek

IF NOT *breathing, give two slow breaths (see ARTIFICIAL RESPIRATION, p.18).*

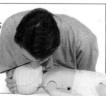

PUT your mouth over baby's mouth and nose

5 Check for pulse

- Place your thumb on the outside of the arm midway between shoulder and elbow
- Use two fingers to feel for a pulse on the inner side of the arm, pressing gently toward the bone
- Feel for five seconds before deciding if pulse is present (a baby's normal pulse is about 120 beats a minute)

CHECK for a pulse on the inner side of upper arm

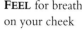
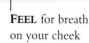
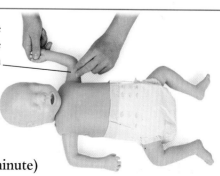
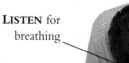
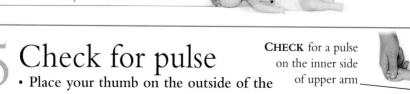

16

6 Act on your findings

Baby unconscious, breathing and pulse present

1 ☎ CALL 911 OR YOUR LOCAL EMS
If you are alone, take your baby with you to the telephone.

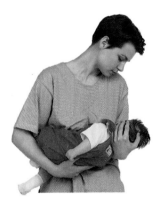

2 Treat any life-threatening injuries such as bleeding (p.46).

3 Cradle your baby in your arms with his head tilted back slightly.

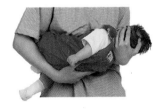

4 Keep your baby in your arms until help arrives and watch closely.

Not breathing but good pulse present

1 Give about 20 breaths of mouth-to-mouth-and-nose respiration for one minute. See p.18.

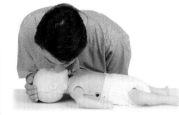

2 ☎ CALL 911 OR YOUR LOCAL EMS
If you are alone, take your baby with you to the telephone.

3 Continue giving mouth-to-mouth-and-nose ventilations.

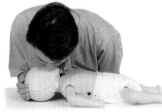

4 Check for pulse every minute (after every 20 breaths).

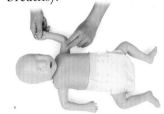

Not breathing, pulse absent

1 Give Cardiopulmonary Resuscitation (CPR) – five chest compressions followed by one breath of mouth-to-mouth-and-nose artificial respiration – repeated for one minute (see p.20).

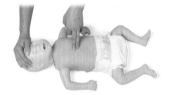
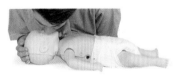

2 ☎ CALL 911 OR YOUR LOCAL EMS
If you are alone, take your baby with you to the telephone.

3 Continue giving Cardiopulmonary Resuscitation (CPR) until help arrives.

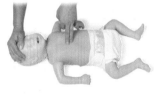
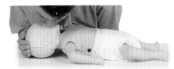

ARTIFICIAL RESPIRATION: BABY

**To be used for an unconscious baby who is not breathing but has a good pulse.
See p.16 to determine unconsciousness and absence of breathing.**

ARTIFICIAL RESPIRATION SUMMARY

UNCONSCIOUS BABY

AIRWAY OPEN

NO BREATHING

GIVE 2 SLOW BREATHS OF **ARTIFICIAL RESPIRATION**

GOOD PULSE PRESENT

GIVE **ARTIFICIAL RESPIRATION** FOR 1 MINUTE

GOOD PULSE PRESENT

☎ CALL 911 OR YOUR LOCAL EMS

CONTINUE **ARTIFICIAL RESPIRATION** UNTIL HELP ARRIVES

18

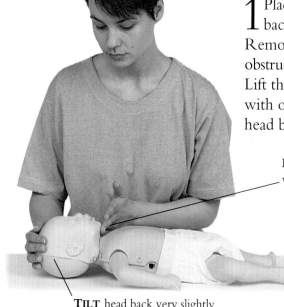

1 Place your baby on his back on a firm surface. Remove any obvious obstruction from the mouth. Lift the point of his chin with one finger and tilt his head back very slightly.

LIFT point of chin with one finger

TILT head back very slightly

2 Seal your lips tightly around your baby's mouth and nose. Breathe gently into the lungs until the chest rises.

BREATHE into the baby's mouth and nose

LET the chest rise

REMOVE your mouth

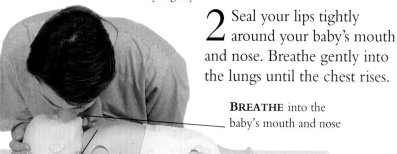

3 Remove your lips and let the chest fall back.

IF *your baby's chest does not rise, check the mouth again. Do not put a finger in the mouth unless you see an obstruction.*

WATCH the chest fall back

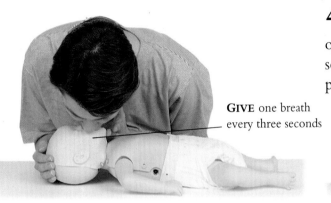

4 Continue to ventilate for one minute, aiming for one slow breath every three seconds (a rate of 20 breaths per minute).

GIVE one breath every three seconds

WATCH chest fall after each breath

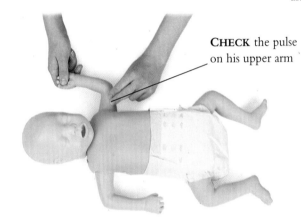

CHECK the pulse on his upper arm

5 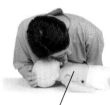 ☎ CALL 911 OR YOUR LOCAL EMS
If you are alone, take your baby with you to the telephone.

19

6 Stop and check that the pulse is still good (see p.16). If it is absent, start Cardiopulmonary Resuscitation (see CPR, p.20).

7 Continue artificial respiration until help arrives. Check the arm pulse every minute. If it is absent, start CPR (see p.20).

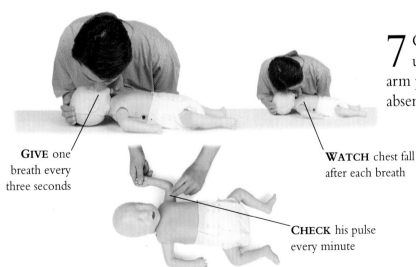

GIVE one breath every three seconds

WATCH chest fall after each breath

CHECK his pulse every minute

CPR (CARDIOPULMONARY RESUSCITATION) : BABY

To be used for an unconscious baby who is not breathing and has no pulse. See p.16 to determine unconsciousness and absence of breathing and pulse.

CPR SUMMARY

UNCONSCIOUS BABY

AIRWAY OPEN

NO BREATHING

GIVE 2 BREATHS OF **ARTIFICIAL RESPIRATION**, See p.18

NO PULSE

CPR – 5 CHEST COMPRESSIONS, 1 BREATH OF ARTIFICIAL RESPIRATION – REPEATED FOR 1 MINUTE

☎ CALL 911 OR YOUR LOCAL EMS

CONTINUE **CPR** UNTIL HELP ARRIVES

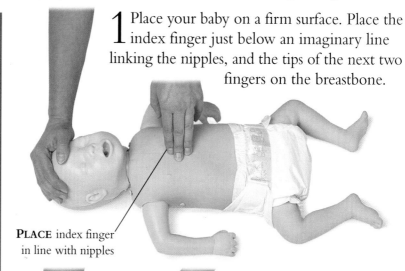

1 Place your baby on a firm surface. Place the index finger just below an imaginary line linking the nipples, and the tips of the next two fingers on the breastbone.

PLACE index finger in line with nipples

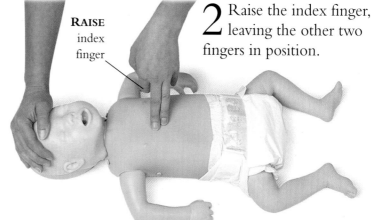

RAISE index finger

2 Raise the index finger, leaving the other two fingers in position.

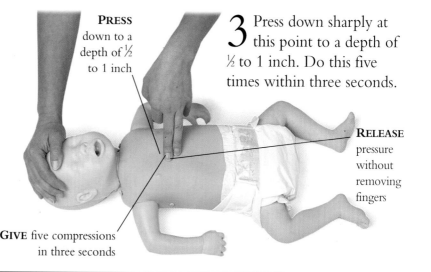

PRESS down to a depth of ½ to 1 inch

3 Press down sharply at this point to a depth of ½ to 1 inch. Do this five times within three seconds.

RELEASE pressure without removing fingers

GIVE five compressions in three seconds

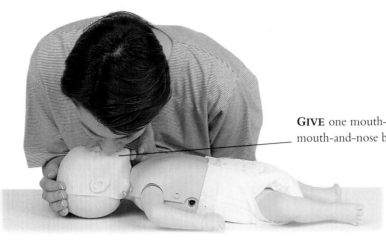

4 Give one full breath of artificial respiration (see p.18).

GIVE one mouth-to-mouth-and-nose breath

Repeat steps 3 and 4 for one minute (about 20 cycles)

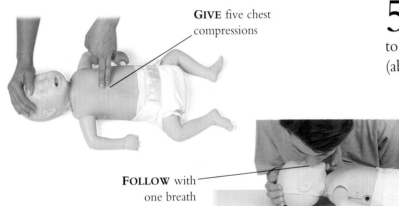

GIVE five chest compressions

5 Continue the cycles of five chest compressions to one breath for one minute (about 20 cycles).

FOLLOW with one breath

21

Repeat CPR cycles until help arrives

6 ☎ CALL 911 OR YOUR LOCAL EMS
If you are alone, take your baby with you to the telephone.

7 Continue giving CPR – five chest compressions followed by one breath of artificial respiration – until the ambulance arrives.

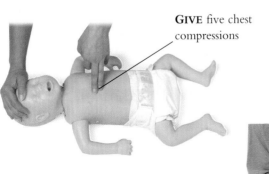

GIVE five chest compressions

FOLLOW with one breath

UNCONSCIOUS CHILD

Assess your child's condition.

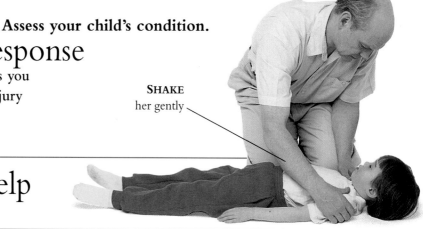

1 Check for response
- Shake her gently, unless you suspect a spinal cord injury
- Call her name
- Pinch her skin

SHAKE her gently

2 Shout for help

3 Open the airway
- Place two fingers under the chin and lift the jaw
- Place other hand on the forehead and tilt the head back
- Look in the mouth and remove any obstruction

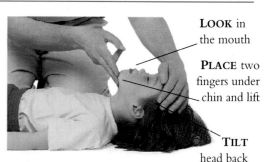

LOOK in the mouth

PLACE two fingers under chin and lift

TILT head back

4 Check for breathing
- Listen for sounds of breathing
- Feel for breath on your cheek
- Look along the chest for movement
- Check for five seconds before deciding if breathing is absent

IF NOT *breathing, give two breaths (see ARTIFICIAL RESPIRATION, p.26).*

CLOSE the child's nose, put your mouth over her mouth, and breathe

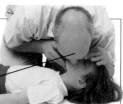

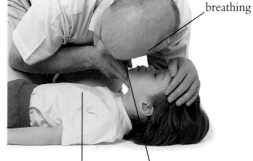

LISTEN for breathing

LOOK for chest movements

FEEL for breath on your cheek

5 Check for pulse
- Keep the head tilted
- Feel for the large muscle at the side of the neck
- Slide two fingers into the groove in front of this muscle
- Press lightly

CHECK for a pulse at her neck

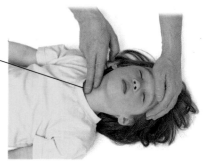

6 Act on your findings

Child unconscious, breathing and pulse present

1 CALL 911 OR YOUR LOCAL EMS

2 Treat any life-threatening injuries such as bleeding (see p.46) or burns (see p.60).

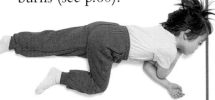

3 Place her in the recovery position (see next page). Do not leave her alone. Keep a check on her breathing and be prepared to resuscitate.

Not breathing but pulse present

1 Give about 20 breaths of mouth-to-mouth respiration for one minute (see p.26).

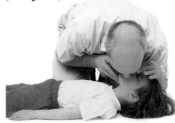

2 CALL 911 OR YOUR LOCAL EMS

3 Continue giving mouth-to-mouth respiration.

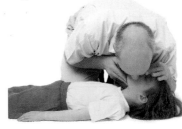

4 Check for pulse every minute (after every 20 breaths).

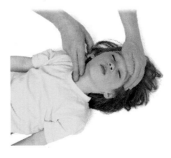

Not breathing, no pulse

1 Give Cardiopulmonary Resuscitation (CPR) – five chest compressions followed by one breath of mouth-to-mouth artificial respiration – repeated for one minute (see p.28).

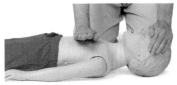

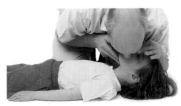

2 CALL 911 OR YOUR LOCAL EMS

3 Continue Cardiopulmonary Resuscitation (CPR) until help arrives.

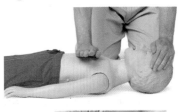

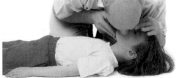

23

RECOVERY POSITION

Put your child in this position if she is unconscious, breathing, and has a pulse
(see p.22), to prevent her choking on her tongue or vomit.

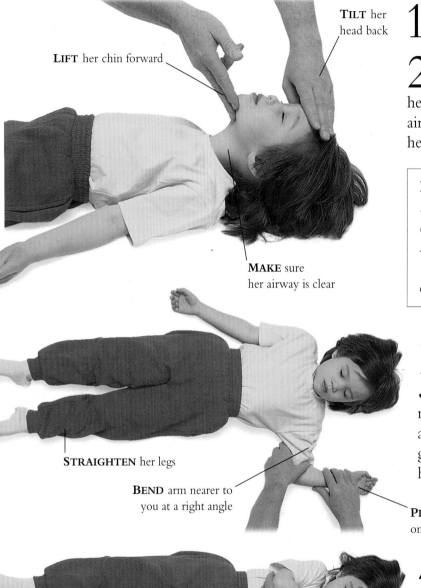

TILT her head back

LIFT her chin forward

MAKE sure her airway is clear

STRAIGHTEN her legs

BEND arm nearer to you at a right angle

PLACE back of her hand on the ground

MOVE farther arm across her chest and bend it

PLACE back of her hand against her cheek

1 ☎ CALL 911 OR YOUR LOCAL EMS.

2 Kneel beside your child. Tilt her head back and lift her chin forward. This keeps her air passages open while you put her in the recovery position.

> **IF** *you suspect BACK AND NECK INJURIES (see pp.73–74) or broken bones (see BONE, JOINT, AND MUSCLE INJURIES, pp.76–84), do not move child. Watch closely – turn only if vomiting.*

3 If necessary, straighten her legs. Bend the arm nearer to you so that it makes a right angle and lay it on the ground, with the palm of the hand upward.

4 Bring her other arm across her chest. Hold the back of her hand against her opposite cheek.

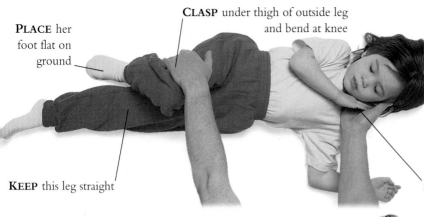

PLACE her foot flat on ground

CLASP under thigh of outside leg and bend at knee

KEEP this leg straight

SUPPORT her hand against her cheek

5 Use your free hand to clasp under the thigh farthest from you. Carefully pull the knee up to bend the leg, leaving the side of the foot flat on the ground.

ROLL her over onto her side by pulling bent leg toward you

KEEP her hand against her cheek

USE your knees to stop her from rolling onto her front

6 Keep your child's hand against her cheek to support her head. At the same time, pull on the thigh of the bent leg to roll her toward you and onto her side.

> **IF** *your child is already lying on her side or is on her front, you will need to adapt the steps when placing her in the recovery position.*

25

> **CHECK** *your child's breathing and pulse frequently while you are waiting for help to arrive.*

ADJUST hand under her cheek

TILT head back again to make sure airway is still open

BEND top leg into a right angle to prevent her from rolling forward

7 Adjust her arm and leg so she cannot fall forward. Tilt her head.

ARTIFICIAL RESPIRATION: CHILD

If an unconscious child is not breathing but still has a pulse, give mouth-to-mouth respiration. See p.22 to determine unconsciousness and absence of breathing.

**ARTIFICIAL
RESPIRATION
SUMMARY**

UNCONSCIOUS CHILD

AIRWAY OPEN

NO BREATHING

GIVE 2 BREATHS OF
**ARTIFICIAL
RESPIRATION**

PULSE PRESENT

GIVE
**ARTIFICIAL
RESPIRATION**
FOR 1 MINUTE

☎ CALL 911 OR
YOUR LOCAL EMS

PULSE PRESENT

CONTINUE
**ARTIFICIAL
RESPIRATION**
UNTIL HELP
ARRIVES

26

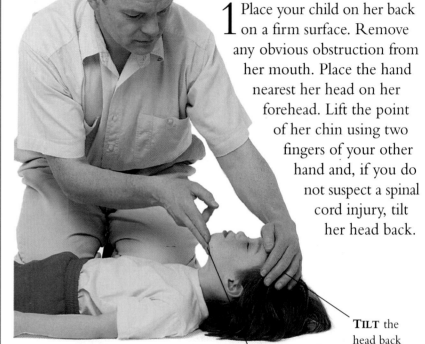

1 Place your child on her back on a firm surface. Remove any obvious obstruction from her mouth. Place the hand nearest her head on her forehead. Lift the point of her chin using two fingers of your other hand and, if you do not suspect a spinal cord injury, tilt her head back.

TILT the head back

LIFT point of chin with two fingers

PINCH nostrils closed

2 Pinch her nostrils closed. Seal your lips round her open mouth. Breathe into the lungs until you see the chest rise.

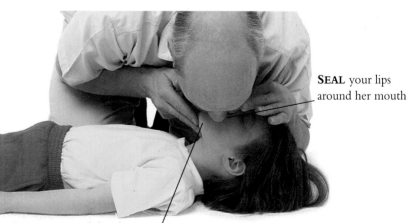

SEAL your lips around her mouth

BREATHE until the chest rises

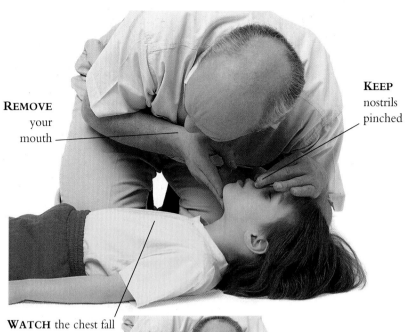

REMOVE your mouth

KEEP nostrils pinched

3 Remove your mouth and let the chest fall. Keep the nostrils pinched.

> **IF** *your child's chest does not rise, reposition the head and chin, then check the mouth again. Do not put your fingers into the mouth unless you see an obstruction.*

WATCH the chest fall

GIVE one breath every three seconds

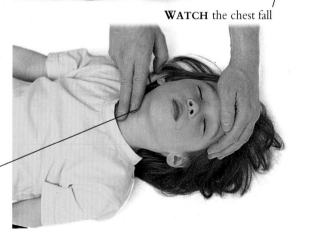

WATCH the chest fall

4 Continue to ventilate for one minute, aiming for a complete breath every three seconds (a rate of 20 per minute).

27

5 ☎ CALL 911 OR YOUR LOCAL EMS

CHECK the pulse at her neck

6 Stop and check that the neck pulse is still present (see p.22). If it is absent, start Cardiopulmonary Resuscitation (see CPR, p.28).

7 Continue artificial respiration until help arrives. Check the neck pulse every minute and if it is absent, begin CPR.

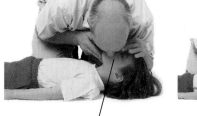

GIVE one breath every three seconds

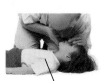

WATCH the chest fall after each breath

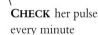

CHECK her pulse every minute

CPR (CARDIOPULMONARY RESUSCITATION) : CHILD

To be used when an unconscious child is not breathing and has no pulse in the neck. See p.22 to determine unconsciousness and absence of breathing and pulse.

CPR SUMMARY

UNCONSCIOUS CHILD

AIRWAY OPEN

NO BREATHING

GIVE 2 BREATHS OF **ARTIFICIAL RESPIRATION**, See p.26

NO PULSE

CPR – 5 CHEST COMPRESSIONS, 1 BREATH OF ARTIFICIAL RESPIRATION, REPEATED FOR 1 MINUTE

CHECK BREATHING AND PULSE

☎ CALL 911 OR YOUR LOCAL EMS

CONTINUE **CPR** IF NEEDED UNTIL HELP ARRIVES

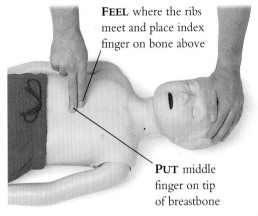

FEEL where the ribs meet and place index finger on bone above

PUT middle finger on tip of breastbone

1 Place your child on her back on a firm surface. Find the point where the ribs meet in the middle line. Place your middle finger on the tip of the breastbone and your index finger on the bone above it.

2 Put the heel of that hand just above where index finger had been.

PLACE hand along breastbone just above where index finger had been

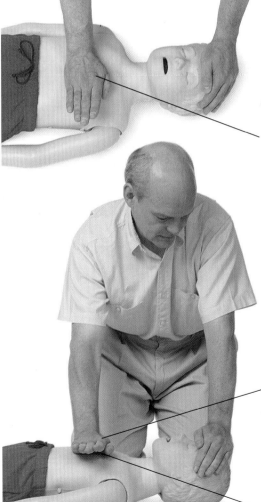

3 Using the heel of that hand, press down sharply at this point to a depth of 1 to 1½ inches. Do this five times within three seconds.

COMPRESS chest five times in three seconds

PRESS down to a depth of 1 to 1½ inches

28

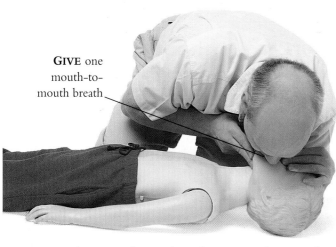

GIVE one mouth-to-mouth breath

4 Give one full breath of artificial respiration about 1½ seconds long (see p.26).

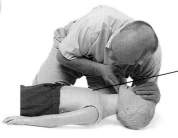

WATCH chest fall

Repeat steps 2 through 4 for one minute (about 20 cycles)

5 Continue the cycles of five chest compressions to one breath for one minute (about 20 cycles).

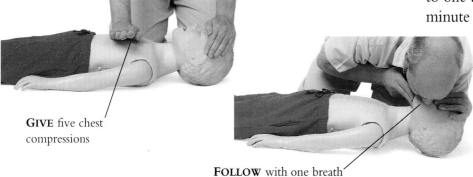

GIVE five chest compressions

FOLLOW with one breath

Repeat CPR cycles until help arrives

6 ☎ CALL 911 OR YOUR LOCAL EMS

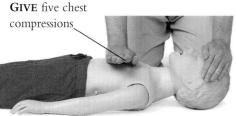

GIVE five chest compressions

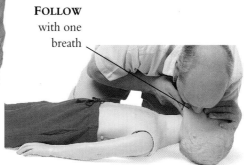

FOLLOW with one breath

DO NOT *stop to make pulse checks unless there are clear signs of life. If pulse and breathing return, place your child in the* RECOVERY POSITION *(see p.24) and watch her carefully until the ambulance arrives.*

7 Continue giving CPR – five chest compressions followed by one breath of artificial respiration – until the ambulance arrives.

29

SHOCK

Recognizing shock Signs of shock include
• *Pale, cold, and sweaty skin that may appear* gray • *A rapid pulse becoming weaker* • *Shallow, fast breathing.*

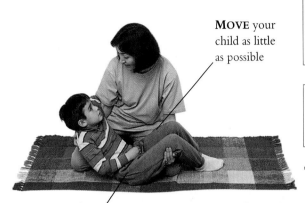

MOVE your child as little as possible

LAY him down, on a blanket, coat, or rug, if possible

> **TRY NOT** *to leave a child in shock unattended. If you can, send someone else to phone for the ambulance while you stay with him.*

> **DO NOT** *give your child anything to drink or eat. If he is thirsty, moisten his lips with water.*

☎ CALL 911 OR YOUR LOCAL EMS

1 Lay your child down flat. Keep his head low as this improves the blood supply to the brain. Turn his head to one side and reassure him. Treat any injury.

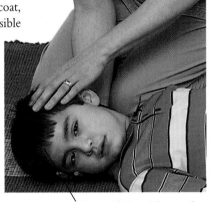

KEEP his head flat on floor and turn it to one side

2 Carefully raise your child's legs 8 to 12 inches and support them with pillows, on a chair, or on a pile of books padded with a cushion.

KEEP his head lower than his chest

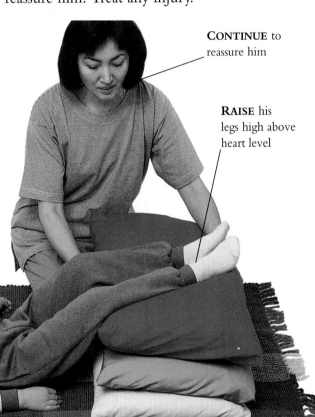

CONTINUE to reassure him

RAISE his legs high above heart level

30

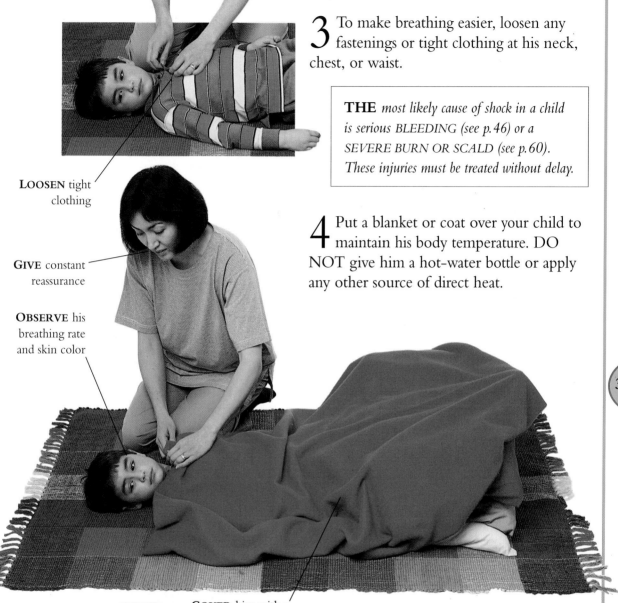

LOOSEN tight
clothing

GIVE constant
reassurance

OBSERVE his
breathing rate
and skin color

COVER him with a
blanket to maintain
body temperature

3 To make breathing easier, loosen any fastenings or tight clothing at his neck, chest, or waist.

> **THE** *most likely cause of shock in a child is serious BLEEDING (see p.46) or a SEVERE BURN OR SCALD (see p.60). These injuries must be treated without delay.*

4 Put a blanket or coat over your child to maintain his body temperature. DO NOT give him a hot-water bottle or apply any other source of direct heat.

31

KEEP checking
his pulse

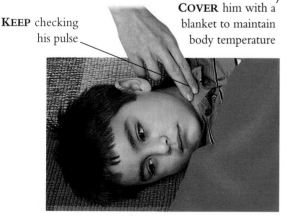

5 Reassure your child. Encourage him to talk or answer questions. This will help you assess his condition. Note any changes and tell the emergency medical technician.

> **IF** *he loses consciousness, assess his condition (see UNCONSCIOUS BABY, p.16; UNCONSCIOUS CHILD, p.22). Be prepared to resuscitate. If he is breathing, place him in the RECOVERY POSITION.*

FEVER CONVULSIONS

Young children under the age of four may develop these convulsions when they have an infection and a high temperature.

Recognizing a convulsion • *He may be flushed and sweating with a very hot forehead* • *His eyes may roll upward, be fixed, or squint* • *His face may look blue* • *He may stiffen and arch his back* • *His fists may clench* • *His arms and legs may jerk.*

1 Undress him down to his diaper. Make sure there is plenty of fresh air in the room without it being cold.

COOL him by taking off his clothes and bedclothes

2 Clear a space around him to protect him from injury. Sponge him with tepid water, starting at his head and working down his body. Do not let him get too cold.

SPONGE him with tepid water until temperature falls

COVER him with a sheet

ROLL him onto his side

3 When the child is cooled, convulsions will stop. Roll him onto his side and try to keep his head tilted back. Cover him with a light blanket or sheet and reassure him. If his temperature rises again, sponge him again. Try not to leave your child unattended.

① CALL A DOCTOR

IF *you can, place him in the RECOVERY POSITION (see p.24) once the convulsions have come to an end.*

32

EPILEPTIC CONVULSIONS

Recognizing epilepsy A seizure progresses through the following stages: • *Sudden falling into unconsciousness, sometimes with a cry* • *Rigidity and arching of back* • *Breathing may cease* • *Jerking movements* • *Froth or bubbles around the mouth, may be blood-stained* • *Bladder or bowel control lost* • *Conscious within a few minutes* • *Dazed feeling* • *Deep sleep may follow.*

Children with a history of epilepsy may have a card or bracelet alerting you to this. A child may have a petit mal seizure before a major one. This can be recognized by a momentary "switching off," some facial twitching, or distracted movements such as lip-smacking. If this happens, reassure the child and arrange to see your doctor.

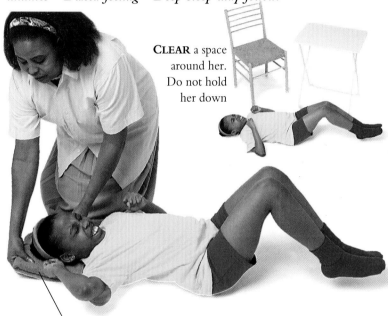

CLEAR a space around her. Do not hold her down

PROTECT her head with soft padding

1 If your child starts to fall, try to catch her and help her to the floor. Clear away objects that she may knock against. Put padding under or around her head. Do not hold her down or try to move her. Don't put anything in her mouth or give her anything to eat or drink.

2 When her convulsions are over, she may be unconscious. Remove any padding, check that the airway is open, and breathing and pulse are present. If breathing, place her in the RECOVERY POSITION (see p.24). Stay with her until she is recovered. She may feel dazed and behave oddly, or she may sleep deeply. ☏ CALL A DOCTOR

Once the convulsions have stopped

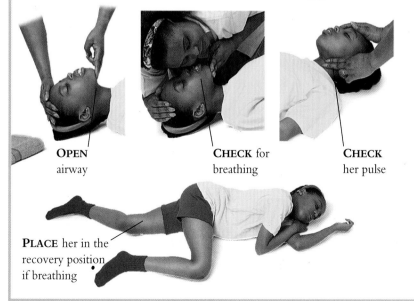

OPEN airway

CHECK for breathing

CHECK her pulse

PLACE her in the recovery position if breathing

IF *your child has never had a seizure before, if she has recurring seizures, or if she remains unconscious for more than ten minutes,* ☎ CALL 911 OR YOUR LOCAL EMS.

33

DIABETIC EMERGENCY

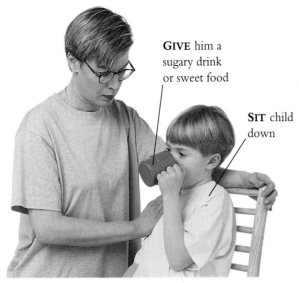

GIVE him a
sugary drink
or sweet food

SIT child
down

Recognizing low blood sugar • *Weakness
or hunger* • *Confused or aggressive behavior*
• *Sweating* • *Very pale face* • *Strong, bounding
pulse* • *Shallow breathing.*

> *A child who is diabetic is likely to be on
> insulin. Even if he seems recovered, a doctor
> should be asked to check the insulin dosage.*

If he improves rapidly after a sweet
drink or food, give him some more
and let him rest. If he does not,
☎ CALL 911 OR
YOUR LOCAL EMS.

An unconscious child

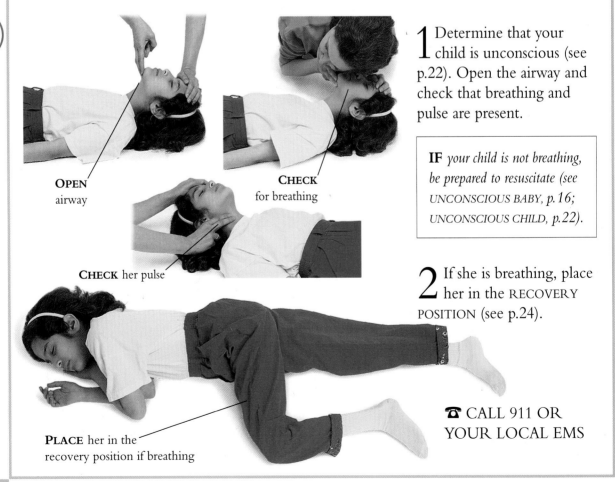

OPEN
airway

CHECK
for breathing

CHECK her pulse

PLACE her in the
recovery position if breathing

1 Determine that your
child is unconscious (see
p.22). Open the airway and
check that breathing and
pulse are present.

> **IF** *your child is not breathing,
> be prepared to resuscitate (see
> UNCONSCIOUS BABY, p.16;
> UNCONSCIOUS CHILD, p.22).*

2 If she is breathing, place
her in the RECOVERY
POSITION (see p.24).

☎ CALL 911 OR
YOUR LOCAL EMS

34

FAINT

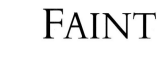

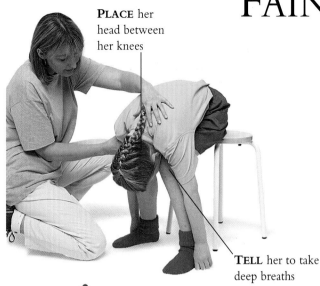

PLACE her head between her knees

TELL her to take deep breaths

Recognizing a faint • *Feeling of weakness, giddiness, and nausea* • *Very pale face* • *Brief loss of consciousness* • *Slow pulse.*

📞 CALL A DOCTOR

1 Tell your child to sit down with her head between her knees. Alternatively, lay her down and raise her legs above the level of her heart, supporting them on a pile of cushions, pillows, or folded blankets about 8 to 12 inches high.

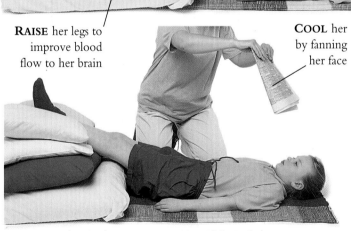

RAISE her legs to improve blood flow to her brain

LOOSEN any tight clothing

COOL her by fanning her face

2 Check that there is no tight clothing around her neck, chest, and waist. Give her plenty of fresh air – open a window, if you are indoors. It may help to fan her face.

3 If she does not regain consciousness, assess her condition (see UNCONSCIOUS BABY, p.16; UNCONSCIOUS CHILD, p.22). Be prepared to resuscitate. If she is breathing, place her in the RECOVERY POSITION (see p.24).
☎ CALL 911 OR YOUR LOCAL EMS

PLACE her in the recovery position if she is slow to regain consciousness

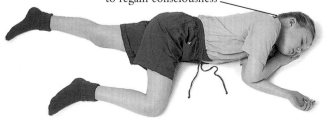

CHOKING: BABY

CHOKING SUMMARY

GIVE 5 SHARP
BACK BLOWS

GIVE 5 CHEST
THRUSTS

CHECK MOUTH

REPEAT CYCLE

5 BACK BLOWS
5 CHEST THRUSTS
CHECK MOUTH

until help arrives
or
obstruction is cleared

36

Recognizing a conscious choking baby • *Breathing is obstructed* • *Face may turn blue* • *Trying to cry but making strange noises, or no sound.*

1 Lay your baby face down with his head low along your forearm. Support his head and shoulders on your hand and give five sharp blows between his shoulders.

DO NOT *shake him or hold him upside down.*

LAY him along your forearm

GIVE five sharp blows on his back

KEEP his head low and support his chin

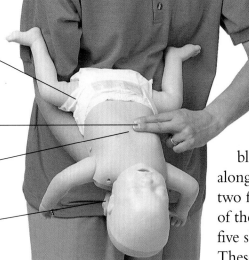

TURN him onto his back

PLACE two fingers on breastbone, just below nipple line

GIVE five sharp downward thrusts

SUPPORT his head and keep it low

2 If back blows fail to clear the blockage, turn him face up along your other arm. Place two fingers on the lower half of the breastbone and give five sharp downward thrusts. These act as artificial coughs.

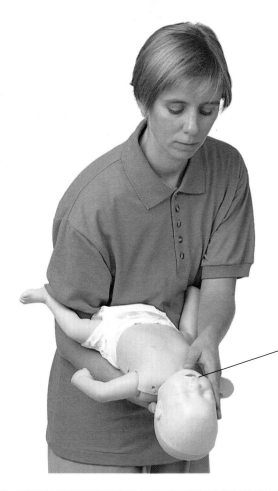

3 Look in his mouth. Put your finger on his tongue to clear the view. Do not put a finger in the mouth unless you can see the obstruction and can hook it out.

If the blockage hasn't cleared, ☎ CALL 911 OR YOUR LOCAL EMS.

LOOK IN his mouth and remove any object you can see

Repeat cycle, following steps 1–3, until help arrives or the obstruction is cleared

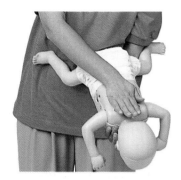

GIVE five back blows

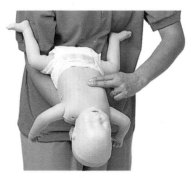

GIVE five chest thrusts

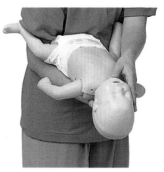

CHECK mouth

IF *your baby loses consciousness, see* UNCONSCIOUS BABY, *p.16. Be prepared to resuscitate.*

CHOKING: CONSCIOUS CHILD

**CONSCIOUS
CHOKING CHILD
SUMMARY**

ENCOURAGE CHILD
TO COUGH

GIVE ABDOMINAL
THRUSTS UNTIL
OBJECT IS EXPELLED

Recognizing a choking child • *Sudden clutching at the throat* • *Child unable to speak or breathe* • *Face may go blue.*

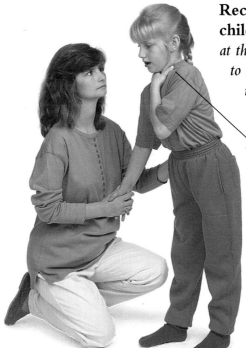

GET her to cough up obstruction if she can

1 Your child may be able to cough up the obsruction on her own. Encourage her to do this, but do not waste time.

38

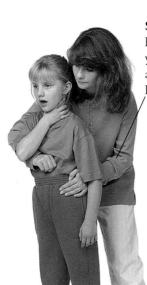

STAND behind her and wrap your arms around her waist

MAKE a fist and grasp it with your other hand

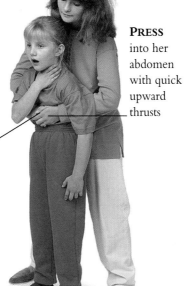

PRESS into her abdomen with quick upward thrusts

IF *she becomes unconscious at any stage, the throat may relax and she may be able to breathe. If she does not breathe, follow the steps on p.39 for an unconscious choking child. Continue until help arrives.*

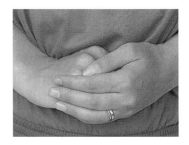

2 Stand or kneel behind her, and wrap your arms around her waist. Make a fist with one hand. Place the thumb side of your fist against the middle of her abdomen, just above her navel.

3 Grasp your fist with the other hand and press into her abdomen with a quick upward thrust.

4 Repeat step 3 until the object is expelled.

UNCONSCIOUS CHILD

If a choking child loses consciousness before you find her, the reason for her unconsciousness may not be obvious.

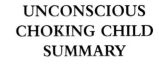

IF a breath will not enter the lungs, retilt her head

1 Determine unconsciousness and check for breathing (see p.22). Attempt to give breaths (see p.26); if the air does not enter the lungs, retilt her head and try again.

☎ CALL 911 OR YOUR LOCAL EMS

2 Straddle the child's legs. Place the heel of one hand just above the navel, with the heel of the other hand on top. Perform 5 abdominal thrusts, pressing inward and upward each time.

POSITION both hands just above the navel, one on top of the other

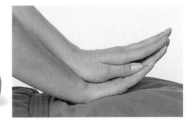

STRADDLE the child's legs

UNCONSCIOUS CHOKING CHILD SUMMARY

ATTEMPT TO GIVE BREATHS

⬇

GIVE 5 ABDOMINAL THRUSTS

⬇

CHECK MOUTH

⬇

REPEAT CYCLE
attempt to give breaths
give 5 abdominal thrusts
check mouth until help arrives
or obstruction is cleared

39

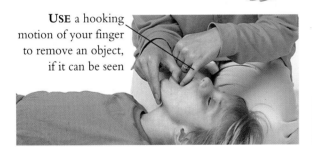

USE a hooking motion of your finger to remove an object, if it can be seen

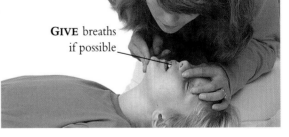

GIVE breaths if possible

3 Look in the mouth, and if you can see an object carefully remove it with a hooking motion, using your smallest finger to avoid pushing the object back down.

DO NOT *put a finger blindly down the throat.*

4 Attempt to give breaths. If you can get air into the child's lungs, continue with artificial respiration (see p.26) even if the object has not been expelled. If you cannot give breaths, repeat the cycle, following steps 2 through 4, until help arrives or the obstruction is cleared.

BREATH HOLDING

Recognizing breath holding Only children under four years of age are likely to do this. • *Your child cries and breathes in but does not breathe out* • *He may go blue in the face and stiff* • *He may become unconscious momentarily.*

Breath holding is the result of rage and frustration. Try to stay calm. Do not shake him or make a fuss. He will usually start breathing spontaneously. If he loses consciousness, see UNCONSCIOUS BABY, p.16; UNCONSCIOUS CHILD, p.22.

☎ CALL 911 OR YOUR LOCAL EMS

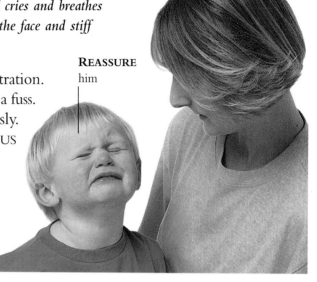

REASSURE him

40

HICCUPS

TELL your child to sit quietly

URGE her to hold her breath for as long as possible

OR

ASK her to hold a paper bag over her mouth and nose

Bending over and drinking from the wrong side of a cup may halt the attack in an older child. **IF** *the hiccups go on for longer than a few hours,* Ⓒ CALL A DOCTOR, *since a long attack can be worrying, tiring, and painful.*

Tell your child to sit still and to hold her breath for as long as she can. Repeat this until the hiccups have gone.
OR
Hold a paper bag over her mouth so that she is rebreathing her own expired air. Get her to breathe in and out for about one minute.

ENCOURAGE her to breathe in and out for one minute or until hiccups stop

SUFFOCATION

This occurs when there is an obstruction over the mouth or nose, a weight on the child's chest or abdomen preventing normal breathing, or because the child is inhaling smoke- or fume-filled air.

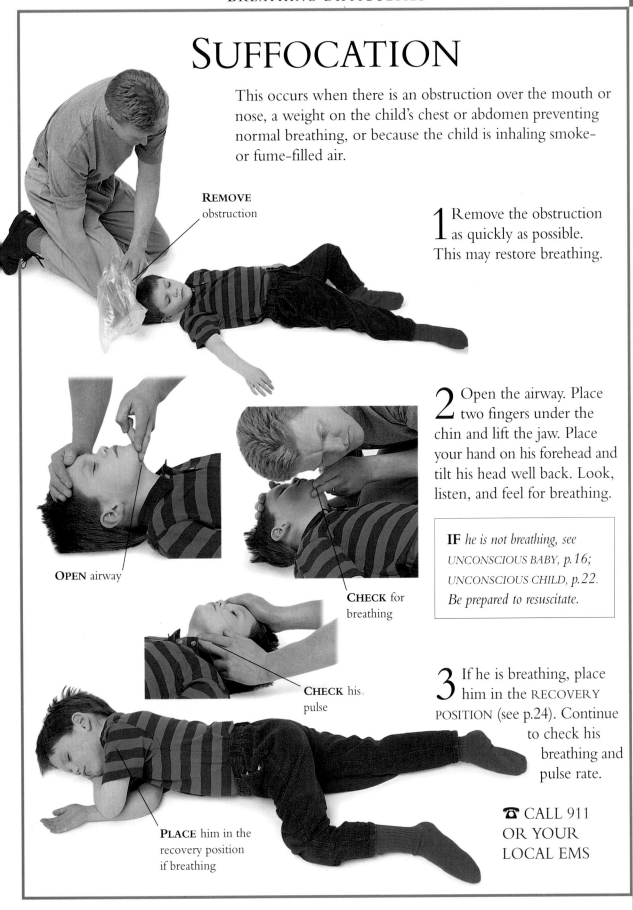

REMOVE obstruction

1 Remove the obstruction as quickly as possible. This may restore breathing.

2 Open the airway. Place two fingers under the chin and lift the jaw. Place your hand on his forehead and tilt his head well back. Look, listen, and feel for breathing.

OPEN airway

CHECK for breathing

> **IF** *he is not breathing, see* UNCONSCIOUS BABY, *p.16;* UNCONSCIOUS CHILD, *p.22.* *Be prepared to resuscitate.*

CHECK his pulse

3 If he is breathing, place him in the RECOVERY POSITION (see p.24). Continue to check his breathing and pulse rate.

PLACE him in the recovery position if breathing

☎ CALL 911 OR YOUR LOCAL EMS

41

STRANGULATION

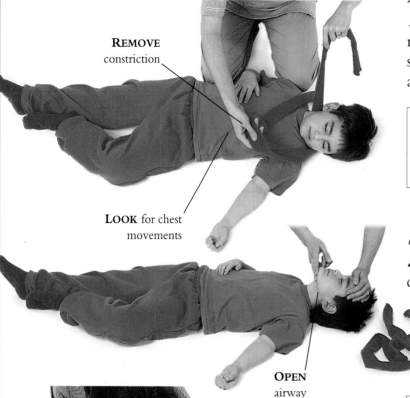

REMOVE constriction

LOOK for chest movements

OPEN airway

CHECK for breathing

CHECK his pulse

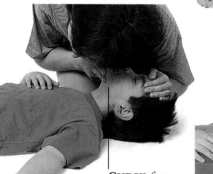

PLACE him in the recovery position if breathing

1 Remove the constriction from around your child's neck without delay. Use scissors or a knife, if they are available, with extreme care.

> **IF** *the child is hanging, support the body while you remove the rope or cord.*

2 Open the airway. Place two fingers under the chin and lift the jaw. Place your hand on his forehead and tilt his head back. Look, listen, and feel for breathing.

> **IF** *he is not breathing, see* UNCONSCIOUS BABY, p.16; UNCONSCIOUS CHILD, p.22. *Be prepared to resuscitate.*

3 If your child is breathing, place him in the RECOVERY POSITION (see p.24). Keep checking his breathing and pulse while you wait.
☎ CALL 911 OR YOUR LOCAL EMS

> **IF** *you suspect* BACK OR NECK INJURIES, *see pp.73-74.*

42

FUME INHALATION

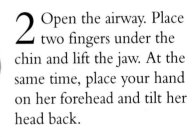

LOOK for chest movements

Fume, gas, and smoke inhalation require urgent medical attention.

☎ CALL 911 OR YOUR LOCAL EMS, AND FIRE DEPARTMENT

1 Carry your child away from the area of danger, without putting yourself at risk.

REMOVE your child into fresh air

IF *your child has any* BURNS, *see p.60.*

OPEN airway

2 Open the airway. Place two fingers under the chin and lift the jaw. At the same time, place your hand on her forehead and tilt her head back.

3 Check for breathing. Feel for breath on your face, look for chest movements, and listen for breathing.

CHECK for breathing

43

IF *your child is not breathing, see* UNCONSCIOUS BABY, *p.16;* UNCONSCIOUS CHILD, *p.22. Be prepared to resuscitate.*

CHECK her pulse

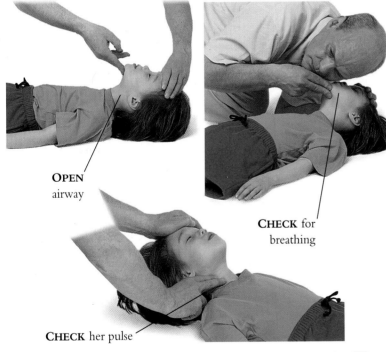

4 If the child is breathing, place her in the RECOVERY POSITION (see p.24) while you wait for help to arrive. Continue to monitor her breathing and pulse.

PLACE her in the recovery position if breathing

CROUP

Recognizing croup This usually occurs at night. It may be alarming, but usually passes quickly. • *Difficulty breathing, particularly inhaling* • *Short, barking cough* • *Crowing or whistling noise.* In a severe attack • *Evidence that the child is using muscles around the nose, neck, and upper arms in his attempts to breathe* • *Blue-tinged skin.*

SIT him up, supporting his back and head

1 Help your child sit up in bed. Prop him up with pillows at his back and head and reassure him.

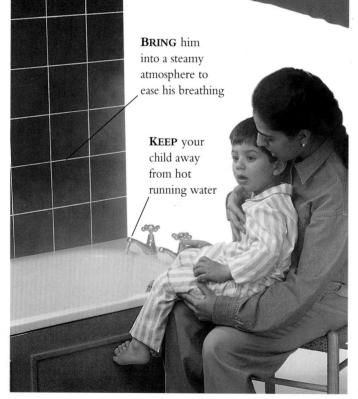

BRING him into a steamy atmosphere to ease his breathing

KEEP your child away from hot running water

2 Create a steamy atmosphere; run hot water into the bath or use a steam vaporizer in an enclosed room. Try to get your child to relax enough to breathe in the steam.

IF *the attack is severe or prolonged,* ☎ CALL 911 OR YOUR LOCAL EMS. *Try to stay calm: if you panic this may alarm your child and worsen the attack.*

44

ASTHMA

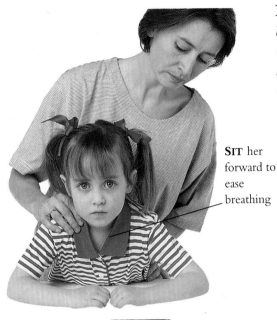

SIT her forward to ease breathing

Recognizing asthma • *Difficulty in breathing often accompanied by coughing* • *Wheezing on breathing out* • *Distress and anxiety* • *Tiredness from labored breathing* • *Bluish tinge to face and lips.*

1 Ensure the room is well-ventilated and smoke-free.

> **IF** *it is a first attack,*
> ℭ CALL A DOCTOR.
> **IF** *the attack is severe or does not respond to medication,*
> ☎ CALL 911 OR YOUR LOCAL EMS.

OR

SIT her on your lap

2 Help your child relax. Sit her down with her arms resting on a table or sit her on your lap. Reassure her since she will be frightened.

> **IF** *your child has special medication, use it immediately in any attack; see below.*

Taking medication

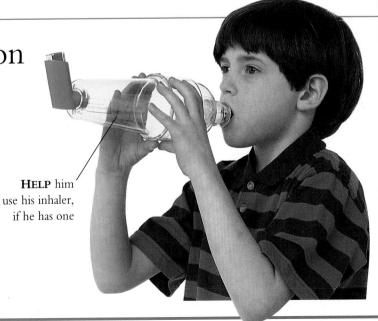

If your child has medication, let him use it. Follow the directions carefully. The attack should ease. If it does not, ☎ CALL 911 OR YOUR LOCAL EMS. Various types of medication are prescribed. Familiarize your child with his medication so that he knows how to use it when he has an attack.

HELP him use his inhaler, if he has one

BLEEDING

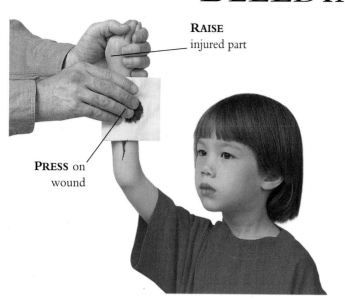

RAISE injured part

PRESS on wound

1 Apply direct pressure to the wound to stop the bleeding. Press a clean pad or handkerchief or, if nothing is available, put the palm of your hand directly on the wound. Raise the injured part above the level of the child's heart.

> **IF** *an object has become stuck in the wound, see* EMBEDDED OBJECT, *p.48.*

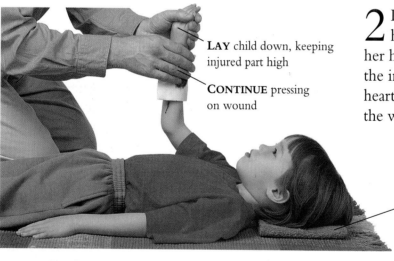

LAY child down, keeping injured part high

CONTINUE pressing on wound

2 Lay your child down, with her head low (put a thin pad under her head for comfort), and keep the injured part raised above the heart. Maintain direct pressure on the wound.

KEEP her head low – use a thin pad for comfort

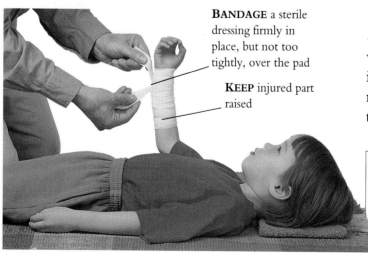

BANDAGE a sterile dressing firmly in place, but not too tightly, over the pad

KEEP injured part raised

3 Cover the wound with a sterile dressing that is larger than the wound. Firmly bandage the dressing in place, keeping the injured part raised. The bandage should not be so tight as to cut off the blood supply.

> **IF** *blood comes through the dressing, bandage another pad firmly on top.*
> **DO NOT** *remove blood-soaked dressing(s).*

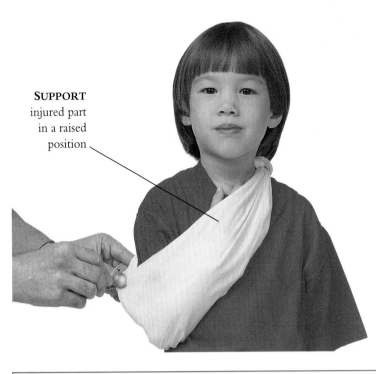

SUPPORT injured part in a raised position

4 When the bleeding is under control, support the injury – for example, with an ELEVATION SLING (see p.111). Check her fingers frequently, for a change in color, temperature, or numbness.

✚ TAKE YOUR CHILD TO THE HOSPITAL

IF *the bleeding persists, follow the treatment for* SHOCK, *below.*
☎ CALL 911 OR YOUR LOCAL EMS

Shock

1 If the bleeding doesn't stop, raise her legs 8 to 12 inches and support them on cushions.

☎ CALL 911 OR YOUR LOCAL EMS

2 Loosen any tight clothing and cover her with a blanket to keep her warm. If she is thirsty, moisten her lips with water, but don't let her drink or eat. (For more on SHOCK, see pp.30–31.)

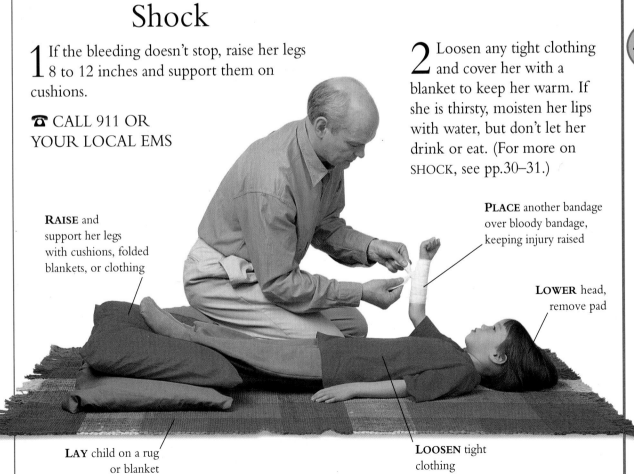

RAISE and support her legs with cushions, folded blankets, or clothing

PLACE another bandage over bloody bandage, keeping injury raised

LOWER head, remove pad

LAY child on a rug or blanket

LOOSEN tight clothing

EMBEDDED OBJECT

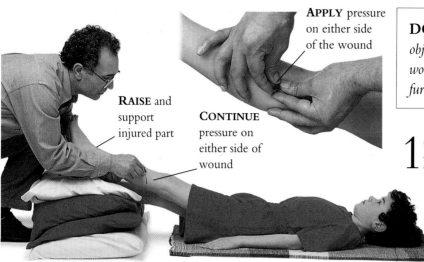

RAISE and support injured part

CONTINUE pressure on either side of wound

APPLY pressure on either side of the wound

DO NOT *try to remove objects that are embedded in a wound since you may cause further damage and bleeding.*

1 Calm your child and lay her down. Apply pressure on either side of the object. Raise injured part above the level of her heart.

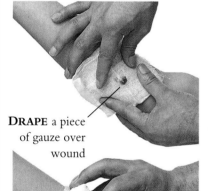

DRAPE a piece of gauze over wound

PLACE padding around the object

BANDAGE over padding

THIS *advanced technique should be performed by the rescuer only if emergency medical services are unavailable or hours away.*

2 Place a piece of gauze over the wound and object to minimize the risk of infection.

3 Use spare bandage rolls to build up padding to the same height as the embedded object.

4 Secure the padding by bandaging over it, being careful not to press on the embedded object.
✚ TAKE YOUR CHILD TO THE HOSPITAL

Bandaging around larger objects

PROTECT object with pads

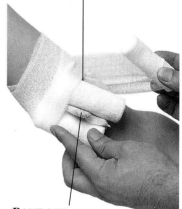

BANDAGE around object

IF *the object is very big, build padding around it and bandage above and below object.*

CUTS AND ABRASIONS

SIT child down

WASH abrasion

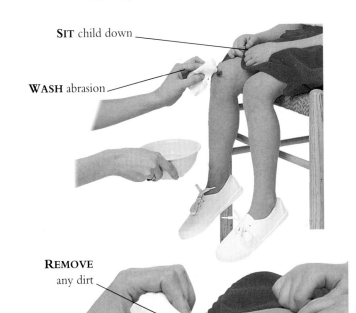

1 Sit your child down and gently wash the abrasion with soap and water using a gauze pad or a washcloth.

REMOVE any dirt

2 Try to remove any particles of dirt or gravel. This may cause a little fresh bleeding.

IF *you cannot remove embedded particles of dirt,* ✚ TAKE YOUR CHILD TO THE HOSPITAL.

49

PRESS clean pad on abrasion

3 Apply pressure with a clean dressing to stop bleeding.

PROTECT abrasion with an adhesive bandage

4 Dress the cut or abrasion with an adhesive bandage that has a pad large enough to cover the wound and the area around it.

DO NOT *cover cuts with cotton or any fluffy material that may stick to the wound and delay healing.*

INFECTED WOUND

COVER
wound with
a clean
dressing

Recognizing an infected wound • *Increasing pain and soreness* • *Swelling, redness, and a feeling of heat around the injury* • *Pus within, or oozing from, the wound* • *Swelling and tenderness of glands in the neck, armpit, or groin* • *Faint red trails on the skin leading to these glands.*

1 Cover the wound with a clean or sterile dressing and then bandage it in place.

BANDAGE
dressing in place

2 Raise and support the infected wound, for example with an ELEVATION SLING (see p.111). Check his fingers frequently for color, temperature, or numbness.

Ⓒ CALL A DOCTOR

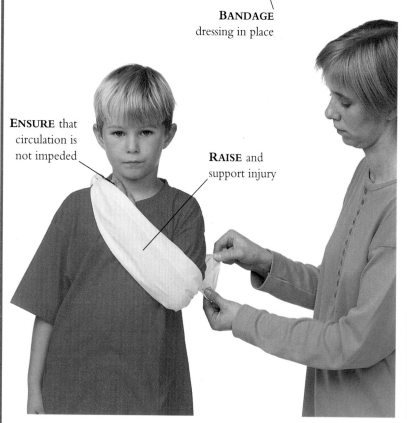

ENSURE that
circulation is
not impeded

RAISE and
support injury

TETANUS *is a dangerous infection that is carried in the air or in the soil. Once present in a wound tetanus germs release toxins (poisons) into the nervous system. It is best prevented through vaccination. Babies receive this as part of their immunization program and a booster is given before starting school.*

50

BLISTERS

CLEAN blister with soap and water

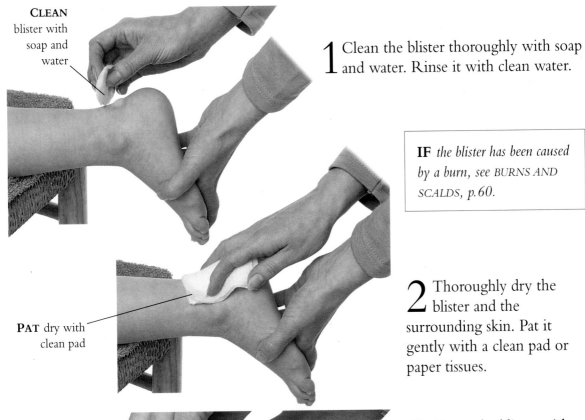

1 Clean the blister thoroughly with soap and water. Rinse it with clean water.

> **IF** *the blister has been caused by a burn, see* BURNS AND SCALDS, *p.60.*

PAT dry with clean pad

2 Thoroughly dry the blister and the surrounding skin. Pat it gently with a clean pad or paper tissues.

COVER with an adhesive bandage, smoothing edges

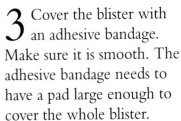

3 Cover the blister with an adhesive bandage. Make sure it is smooth. The adhesive bandage needs to have a pad large enough to cover the whole blister.

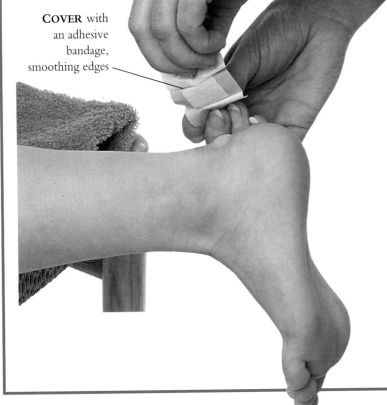

> **IF** *the blister is very large, cover it with a clean dressing and hold it in place with adhesive tape or a bandage. Never deliberately break a blister since this can cause it to become infected.*

EYE WOUND

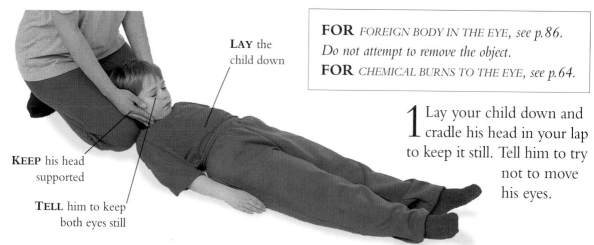

LAY the child down

KEEP his head supported

TELL him to keep both eyes still

FOR *FOREIGN BODY IN THE EYE, see p.86.*
Do not attempt to remove the object.
FOR *CHEMICAL BURNS TO THE EYE, see p.64.*

1 Lay your child down and cradle his head in your lap to keep it still. Tell him to try not to move his eyes.

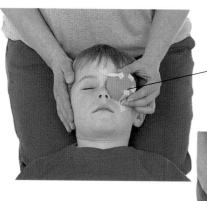

COVER injured eye with bottom of a paper cup and tape in place

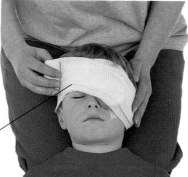

BANDAGE cup to secure it

2 Reassure your child. Then cover the injury, avoiding any pressure on the eye. Use a paper or styrofoam cup, cut 1½ in from the bottom. Tape cup firmly, but gently, over the injured eye. Then bandage in place.

DO NOT *touch the injured eye.*

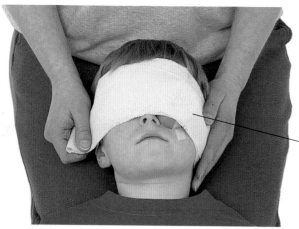

COVER both eyes with bandage

3 Bandage both eyes, to keep blood, fluid, and dirt out of the uninjured eye.

☎ CALL 911 OR YOUR LOCAL EMS
Keep him lying on his back.

52

NOSEBLEED

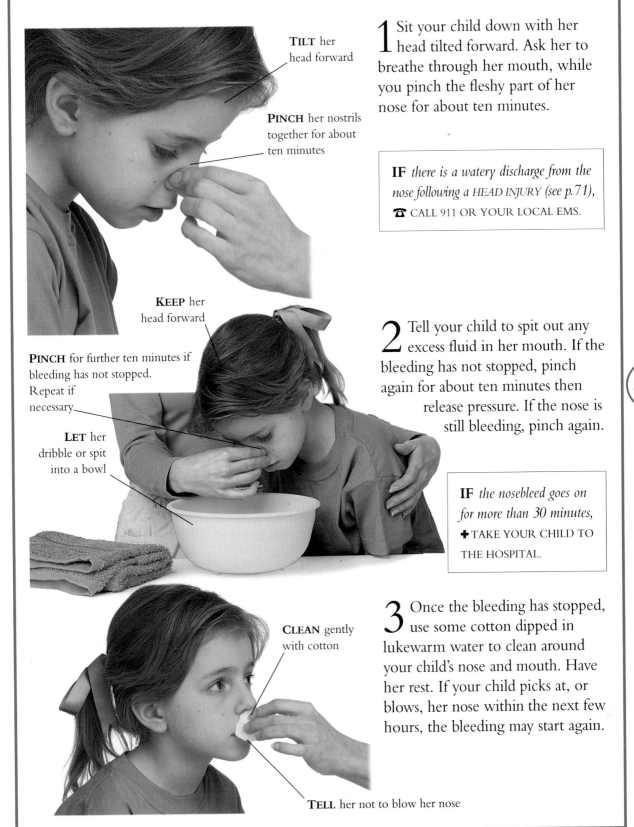

TILT her head forward

PINCH her nostrils together for about ten minutes

KEEP her head forward

PINCH for further ten minutes if bleeding has not stopped. Repeat if necessary

LET her dribble or spit into a bowl

CLEAN gently with cotton

TELL her not to blow her nose

1 Sit your child down with her head tilted forward. Ask her to breathe through her mouth, while you pinch the fleshy part of her nose for about ten minutes.

IF *there is a watery discharge from the nose following a HEAD INJURY (see p.71),* ☎ CALL 911 OR YOUR LOCAL EMS.

2 Tell your child to spit out any excess fluid in her mouth. If the bleeding has not stopped, pinch again for about ten minutes then release pressure. If the nose is still bleeding, pinch again.

IF *the nosebleed goes on for more than 30 minutes,* ✚ TAKE YOUR CHILD TO THE HOSPITAL.

3 Once the bleeding has stopped, use some cotton dipped in lukewarm water to clean around your child's nose and mouth. Have her rest. If your child picks at, or blows, her nose within the next few hours, the bleeding may start again.

53

EAR

Bleeding from inside the ear

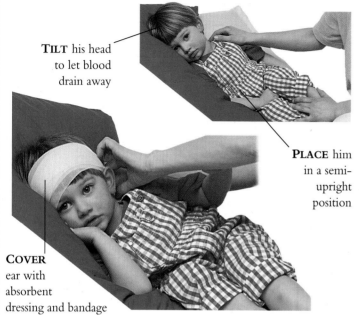

TILT his head to let blood drain away

PLACE him in a semi-upright position

COVER ear with absorbent dressing and bandage

1 Help your child into a semi-upright position, with his head tilted toward the injured side, to allow blood to drain away.

2 Put an absorbent dressing over the ear and bandage it lightly in place. Do not plug the ear.

✆ CALL A DOCTOR

IF *the bleeding follows a* HEAD INJURY *(see p. 71) and/or the fluid draining from the ear is thin and watery, do not bandage.*

☎ CALL 911 OR YOUR LOCAL EMS

External bleeding

1 Gently pinch the wound with a piece of gauze, pressing for about ten minutes.

2 Cover her ear with a sterile dressing and lightly bandage it in place.

✆ CALL A DOCTOR

PRESS on wound over a clean pad for about ten minutes

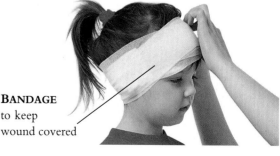

BANDAGE to keep wound covered

IF *the injury is caused by an earring being ripped out, your child may need stitches.*

✚ TAKE YOUR CHILD TO THE HOSPITAL

MOUTH INJURY

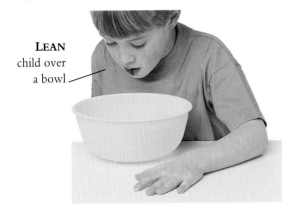

LEAN child over a bowl

> **DO NOT** *wash out his mouth because this may disturb a blood clot.*

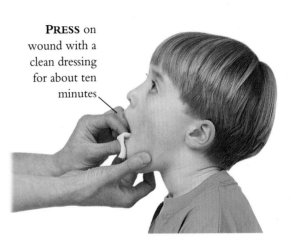

PRESS on wound with a clean dressing for about ten minutes

1 Sit your child down, with his head over a bowl into which he can dribble the blood.

2 Place a dressing over the wound and pinch it between your thumb and forefinger, maintaining the pressure for about ten minutes.

Knocked-out tooth

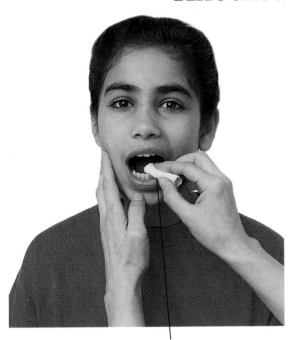

HOLD a pad over the tooth socket

> **AN "ADULT" TOOTH** *may be replanted. Do not clean it. Put the tooth in milk.*
> ✚ TAKE YOUR CHILD TO THE DENTIST

1 Place a dressing over the tooth socket, making sure that the dressing is higher than the adjacent teeth so that your child can bite on it.

2 Ask your child to sit down with her hand supporting her jaw. Tell her to bite hard on the dressing. A younger child may need you to hold the dressing in place.

> **BABY TEETH** *are not replanted, but find the missing tooth to ensure that it has not been inhaled or swallowed. A dentist should check the gum.*

AMPUTATION

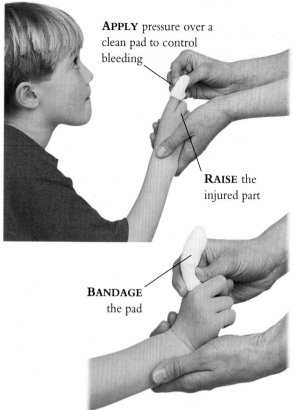

APPLY pressure over a clean pad to control bleeding

RAISE the injured part

BANDAGE the pad

1 Control the blood loss by pressing firmly on the injury with a sterile dressing. Raise the injured part above the level of your child's heart.

> **DO NOT** *use a tourniquet.*

2 Bandage or tape the dressing firmly in place. You can cover a finger with a gauze finger bandage.

☎ CALL 911 OR YOUR LOCAL EMS and tell the dispatcher it is an amputation.

> **YOU** *may need to treat your child for* SHOCK, *see p.30, and* BLEEDING, *p.46.*

Care of the amputated part

It is sometimes possible to "replant" an amputated part using microsurgery. The sooner both the child and the severed part reach the hospital, the better. **NEVER** *wash the severed part or allow it to come into direct contact with the ice.* **DO NOT** *apply cotton to any raw surface.*

2 Wrap the bag in a soft fabric, such as a cotton handkerchief or gauze.

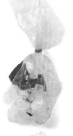

3 Put a plastic bag filled with ice cubes around the fabric. This helps preserve the severed part.

1 Wrap the severed part in plastic wrap or a plastic bag.

4 Put the whole package in another bag or container. Mark with the time of injury and the child's name. Give it to the ambulance attendant.

INTERNAL BLEEDING

Suspect this when signs of shock develop without obvious blood loss.

Recognizing internal bleeding • *Pale, cold, and sweaty skin that may appear blue or gray* • *A rapid pulse becoming weaker* • *Shallow, fast breathing* • *Restlessness, yawning, and sighing* • *Thirst* • *Possible loss of consciousness.* After violent injury, there may be • *"Pattern bruising" at the site of injury with marks from clothes or crushing objects* • *Bleeding from orifices – note what it looks like and try to take a sample to the hospital.*

See HEAD INJURY (p.71), SHOCK (p.30).

☎ CALL 911 OR YOUR LOCAL EMS

> **IF** *your child loses consciousness, assess his condition (see UNCONSCIOUS BABY, p.16; UNCONSCIOUS CHILD, p.22). Be prepared to resuscitate.*

Lay her down with her legs raised 8 to 12 inches. Check her breathing and pulse.

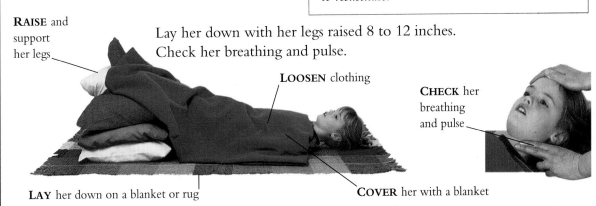

RAISE and support her legs

LOOSEN clothing

CHECK her breathing and pulse

LAY her down on a blanket or rug

COVER her with a blanket

CRUSH INJURY

☎ CALL 911 OR YOUR LOCAL EMS

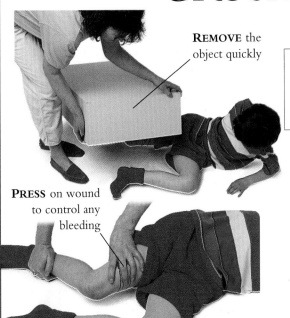

REMOVE the object quickly

PRESS on wound to control any bleeding

> **IF** *the child has been crushed for more than ten minutes, do not remove the object, since this increases the risk of shock and further internal injury. Reassure your child.*

1 If the accident has just happened, remove the heavy object quickly.

2 Control any bleeding by pressing firmly on the wound, with a clean pad or your hand.

> **IF** *you suspect broken bones, support the injury with padding, but do not move your child until help arrives. Watch for signs of SHOCK (see above and p.30).*

CHEST WOUND

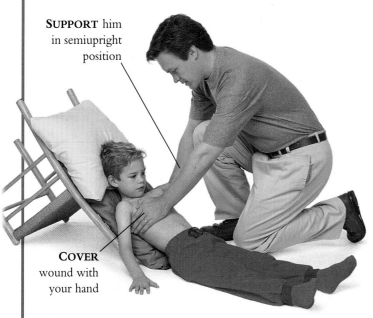

SUPPORT him in semiupright position

COVER wound with your hand

THIS advanced technique should be performed by the rescuer only if emergency medical services are unavailable or hours away.

A chest wound may cause severe internal damage. The lungs are particularly vulnerable, and breathing problems, shock, and collapsed lungs may follow an injury. It is important to make an airtight seal over the wound to prevent air from entering the cavity.

☎ CALL 911 OR YOUR LOCAL EMS

1 Cover the wound with the palm of your hand and support your child in a semiupright position.

2 With your child supported, cover the wound with a sterile dressing and tape it in place.

3 Create an airtight seal by covering the pad with a piece of plastic wrap, secured in place with adhesive tape. Leave one corner untaped to permit exhaled air to escape.

4 Incline your child toward his injured side, supported on cushions.

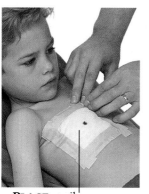

PLACE sterile dressing over wound

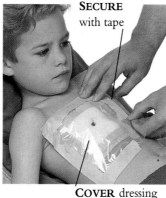

SECURE with tape

COVER dressing with plastic wrap

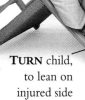

REASSURE him

TURN child, to lean on injured side

IF your child loses consciousness, assess his condition (see UNCONSCIOUS BABY, p.16; UNCONSCIOUS CHILD, p.22). Be prepared to resuscitate. If breathing, place him in the RECOVERY POSITION (see p.24), lying on his injured side. Check for signs of SHOCK (see p.30).

ABDOMINAL WOUND

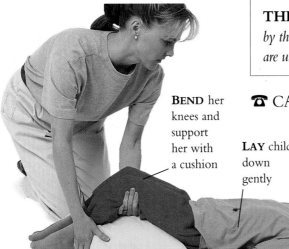

> **THIS** *advanced technique should be performed by the rescuer only if emergency medical services are unavailable or hours away.*

BEND her knees and support her with a cushion

LAY child down gently

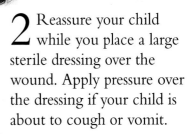

☎ CALL 911 OR YOUR LOCAL EMS

1 Lay your child down and place a cushion or pillow under her knees to ease the strain on her abdomen. Loosen any tight clothing.

COVER wound with dressing

2 Reassure your child while you place a large sterile dressing over the wound. Apply pressure over the dressing if your child is about to cough or vomit.

> **IF** *part of the intestine is showing, cover it with a polyethylene bag or plastic wrap before dressing the wound.*

TAPE dressing in place

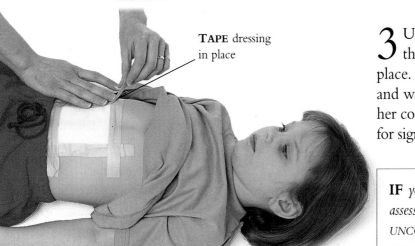

3 Use adhesive tape to secure the dressing lightly in place. Continue to reassure her and watch for any change in her condition; look particularly for signs of SHOCK (see p.30).

> **IF** *your child loses consciousness, assess her condition (see* UNCONSCIOUS BABY, *p.16;* UNCONSCIOUS CHILD, *p.22). Be prepared to resuscitate.*

59

BURNS AND SCALDS

For information on dealing with fires, see
ACTION IN AN EMERGENCY, p.11.

DO NOT *remove any clothing or material that may be sticking to the burned area because this may cause further damage to the skin.*

IF *no water is available, use another cool liquid such as milk.*

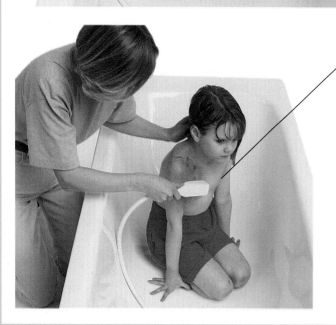

COOL burn with cool water for at least ten minutes

✚ TAKE YOUR CHILD TO THE HOSPITAL OR
☎ CALL 911 OR YOUR LOCAL EMS

1 To stop the burning process and relieve pain, cool the burn with cool water for at least ten minutes.

DO NOT *immerse young children in cold water since this can cause hypothermia.*

REMOVE cooled clothing and cool injury again

2 Once cooled, remove clothing from the burned area and, if the pain persists, cool again. Cut around any material sticking to the skin. Remove restrictive clothing from the area of a burn before the burn area begins to swell.

DO NOT *touch the burn or burst any blisters.*

60

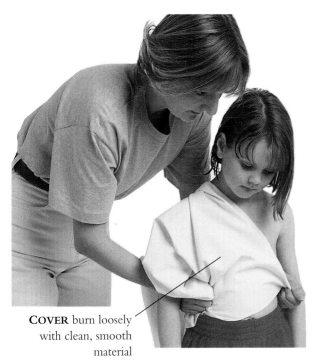

COVER burn loosely
with clean, smooth
material

3 Cover the burn with clean, smooth
material to protect it from infection.
You can use a clean sheet or pillow case.
The dressing does not need to be secured.
Do not apply lotions, fat, or ointment.

> **DO NOT** *give her anything to eat or drink;*
> *watch for signs of SHOCK (see p.30).*

> **IF** *your child loses consciousness, assess her*
> *condition (see UNCONSCIOUS BABY, p.16;*
> *UNCONSCIOUS CHILD, p.22). Be prepared to*
> *resuscitate. If breathing, place her in the*
> *RECOVERY POSITION (p.24).*

Alternative dressings To
dress a burned hand or foot you
can use a plastic bag. Secure
this with an adhesive bandage
around the bag, not the skin.

PROTECT
with clean
plastic bag

61

Burns to the mouth and throat

Burns in this area are very dangerous
because they cause swelling and
inflammation of the air passages, giving
a serious risk of suffocation. Act
quickly. If necessary, loosen clothing
from around his neck. Give him
cool water to sip.

☎ CALL 911 OR YOUR LOCAL EMS

> **IF** *he develops breathing difficulties,*
> *assess his condition (see UNCONSCIOUS*
> *BABY, p.16; UNCONSCIOUS CHILD,*
> *p.22). Be prepared to resuscitate.*

GIVE him
cool water
to sip

LOOSEN clothing
around his neck

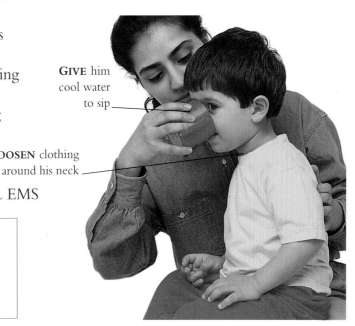

ELECTRICAL BURN

An electric shock from a low-voltage source can result in burns. These may occur at both the point of entry and the point of exit of an electrical current. See ELECTRICAL INJURY (p.12), SHOCK (p.30).

> **DO NOT** *touch your child until you are sure the electrical current is switched off.*

> **IF** *your child loses consciousness, assess her condition (see* UNCONSCIOUS BABY, *p.16;* UNCONSCIOUS CHILD, *p.22). Be prepared to resuscitate. If breathing, place her in the* RECOVERY POSITION *(see p.24).*

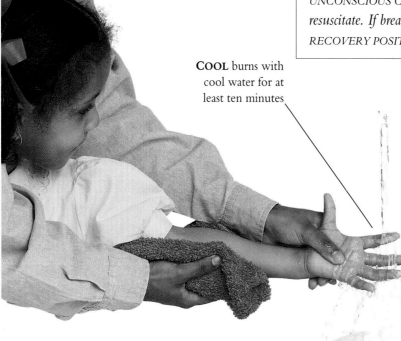

COOL burns with cool water for at least ten minutes

1 Hold the injured area under cool, running water for at least ten minutes to cool the burn.

2 Protect the burn by covering it with clean, smooth material or with a plastic bag, held or taped in place.

✚ TAKE YOUR CHILD TO THE HOSPITAL

COVER with a clean plastic bag

CHEMICAL BURN TO SKIN

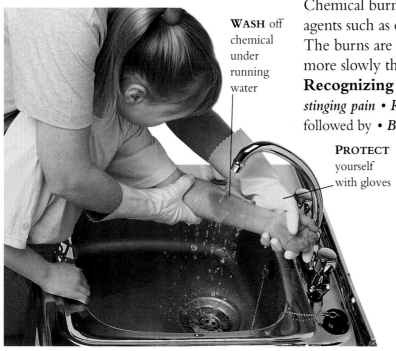

WASH off chemical under running water

PROTECT yourself with gloves

Chemical burns can be caused by household agents such as oven cleaner or paint thinners. The burns are serious but signs develop more slowly than for thermal burns.
Recognizing chemical burns • *Fierce, stinging pain* • *Redness or skin discoloration,* followed by • *Blistering and peeling.*

1 Wash away all traces of the chemical by holding the affected area under plenty of running water.

> **NOTE** *the name of the substance that caused the burn. Wear protective rubber gloves, and beware of fumes. See FUME INHALATION (p.43) and SWALLOWED CHEMICALS (p.65).*

63

Removing clothes

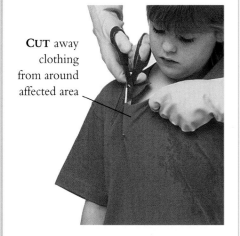

CUT away clothing from around affected area

2 Cut off clothing from the affected area, unless you can slip it off without touching other parts of the body. Avoid cutting through the affected area – cut around it instead.

COVER burn loosely with clean material

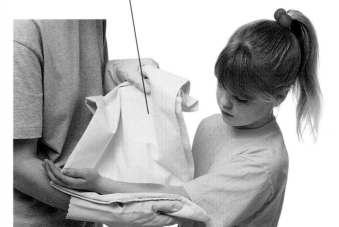

3 Loosely cover the burn with clean, smooth material, such as a pillowcase. This avoids constriction when the wound swells. You can wet the pillowcase to cool and soothe the burn.

✚ TAKE YOUR CHILD TO THE HOSPITAL

CHEMICAL BURNS TO EYE

Splashes of chemicals in the eye can cause scarring or even blindness.

Recognizing chemical burns to the eye
- *Fierce pain in the eye* • *Difficulty opening the eye*
- *Redness and swelling in and around the eye*
  - *Very watery eye.*

WASH eye with cool water for at least ten minutes

LET water drain away

> **DO NOT** *let your child rub her eye.*

> **THE EYE** *will be shut in spasm and pain, so gently pull the eyelids open.*

USE a jug, if this is easier

BE careful not to splash water in her face

1 Hold your child over a basin, with the good eye uppermost, and gently run cool water over the contaminated eye for at least ten minutes. Wear protective gloves. Make sure that both sides of the eyelid are thoroughly washed and that the water drains away from her face. You may find it easier to use a jug. Avoid splashing the good eye with contaminated water.

COVER injured eye with paper cup and bandage in place

2 When the injured eye is thoroughly washed, cover it, avoiding any pressure on the eye. Use a paper or styrofoam cup, cut 1½ in from the bottom, and place the base over the eye. Secure it with tape, then bandage it in place.

✚ TAKE YOUR CHILD TO THE HOSPITAL

64

SWALLOWED CHEMICALS

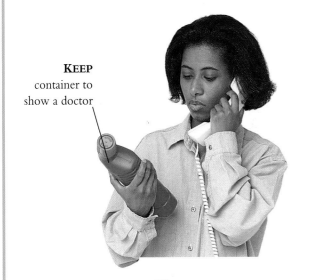

KEEP container to show a doctor

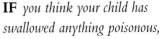

IF *you think your child has swallowed anything poisonous,*
☠CALL YOUR POISON CONTROL CENTER

1 Find out what chemical your child swallowed; this will help determine the correct medical treatment.
☠ CALL YOUR POISON CONTROL CENTER

WASH your child's lips and mouth gently

2 Wipe away any residual chemical around the mouth and face. Remove any contaminated clothing (see p.63).

DO NOT *try to make your child vomit since this can cause further harm.*

3 Give her frequent sips of cool water or milk if her lips are burned or discolored.

✚ TAKE YOUR CHILD TO THE HOSPITAL OR
☎ CALL 911 OR YOUR LOCAL EMS

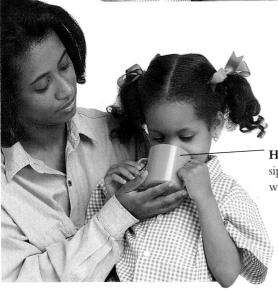

HELP her take sips of cool water or milk

IF *your child loses consciousness, assess her condition (see UNCONSCIOUS BABY, p.16; UNCONSCIOUS CHILD, p.22). Be prepared to resuscitate. If breathing, place her in the RECOVERY POSITION (see p.24).*

65

DRUG POISONING

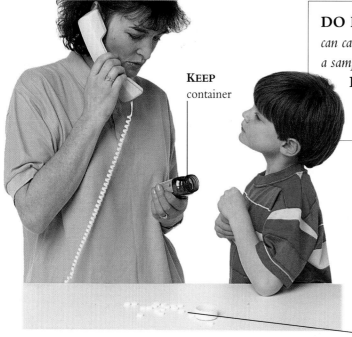

KEEP container

DO NOT *make your child vomit since it can cause further harm. If he does vomit, keep a sample to show the doctor.*
    DO NOT *give fluids since this will help dissolve the drugs and hasten absorption into the body.*

☠ CALL YOUR POISON CONTROL CENTER
Talk calmly to your child and try to find out when he took the pills, and how many he swallowed. Examine the label on the medicine bottle and give the information to your doctor.

COUNT how many pills are left

If the child is unconscious

☎ CALL 911 OR YOUR LOCAL EMS

CLEAR his mouth, if necessary

1 Open his mouth. Hook out with a finger any drugs that you can see.

TRY *to find out what drugs he has taken and how much he has swallowed.*

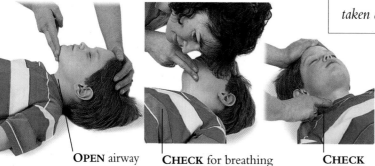

OPEN airway   **CHECK** for breathing   **CHECK** his pulse

PLACE him in recovery position if breathing

2 Open his airway. Check his breathing and pulse (see UNCONSCIOUS BABY, p.16; UNCONSCIOUS CHILD, p.22). Be prepared to resuscitate. If he is breathing, place him in the RECOVERY POSITION (see p.24). Stay with him until help arrives.

ALCOHOL POISONING

EVEN *a small amount of alcohol may harm a young child.*

Recognizing alcohol poisoning
• *A strong smell of alcohol* • *Flushed and moist face* • *Slurred speech* • *Staggering* • *Deep noisy breathing* • *Nausea* • *Bounding pulse.*

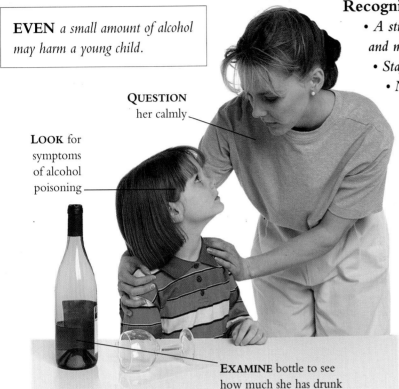

QUESTION her calmly

LOOK for symptoms of alcohol poisoning

EXAMINE bottle to see how much she has drunk

☠ CALL YOUR POISON CONTROL CENTER

Allow your child to rest where you can watch over her. Place a bowl nearby in case she vomits. If she falls asleep, check her to make sure she can be easily roused. If she is very drowsy, or seems unconscious, see below.

67

If the child is unconscious

☎ CALL 911 OR YOUR LOCAL EMS

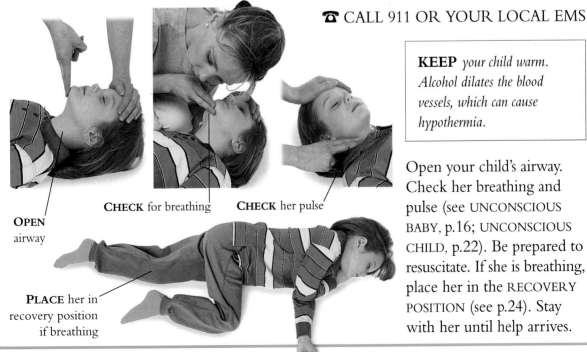

KEEP *your child warm. Alcohol dilates the blood vessels, which can cause hypothermia.*

OPEN airway

CHECK for breathing

CHECK her pulse

PLACE her in recovery position if breathing

Open your child's airway. Check her breathing and pulse (see UNCONSCIOUS BABY, p.16; UNCONSCIOUS CHILD, p.22). Be prepared to resuscitate. If she is breathing, place her in the RECOVERY POSITION (see p.24). Stay with her until help arrives.

PLANT POISONING

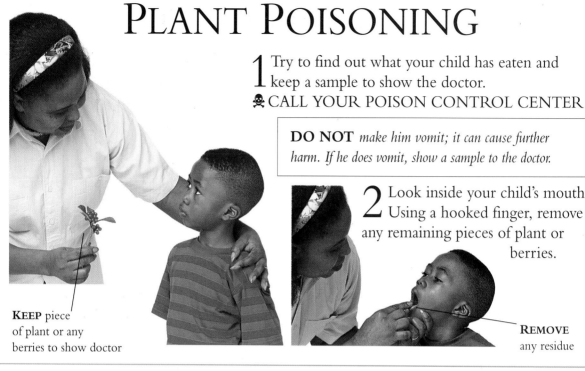

1 Try to find out what your child has eaten and keep a sample to show the doctor.
☠ CALL YOUR POISON CONTROL CENTER

DO NOT *make him vomit; it can cause further harm. If he does vomit, show a sample to the doctor.*

2 Look inside your child's mouth. Using a hooked finger, remove any remaining pieces of plant or berries.

KEEP piece of plant or any berries to show doctor

REMOVE any residue

If the child is unconscious

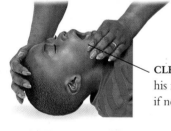

CLEAR his mouth, if necessary

1 Open his mouth. Hook out with a finger any pieces of plant that you can see.

☎ CALL 911 OR YOUR LOCAL EMS

OPEN airway

CHECK for breathing

CHECK his pulse

2 Open his airway. Check his breathing and pulse (see UNCONSCIOUS BABY, p.16; UNCONSCIOUS CHILD, p.22). Be prepared to resuscitate. If he is breathing, place him in the RECOVERY POSITION (see p.24). Stay with him until the ambulance arrives.

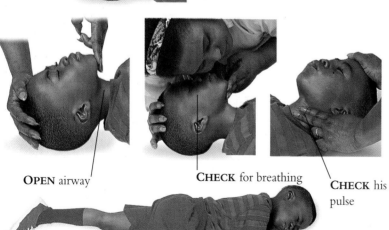

PLACE him in recovery position if breathing

SCALP WOUND

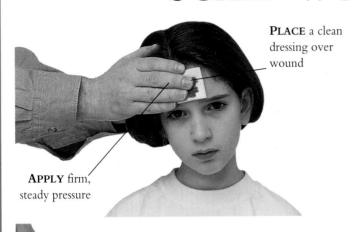

PLACE a clean dressing over wound

APPLY firm, steady pressure

1 Cover the injury with a clean or sterile dressing that is larger than the wound. Scalp wounds can bleed profusely, so press firmly on the pad and the wound to control the bleeding. Place another pad on top, if the first becomes too wet, but do not remove the first dressing. Keeping pressing.

BANDAGE pad in place

2 Bandage the dressing firmly in place. If the bleeding continues, apply pressure again with your hand.

SECURE bandage firmly but not too tightly

> **IF** *the wound has been caused by a blow to the head,*
> ✚ TAKE YOUR CHILD TO THE HOSPITAL *(see also CONCUSSION, p.70; SKULL FRACTURE, p.71).*

3 Lay your child to down with her head and shoulders slightly raised. Watch for signs of shock (see p.30).

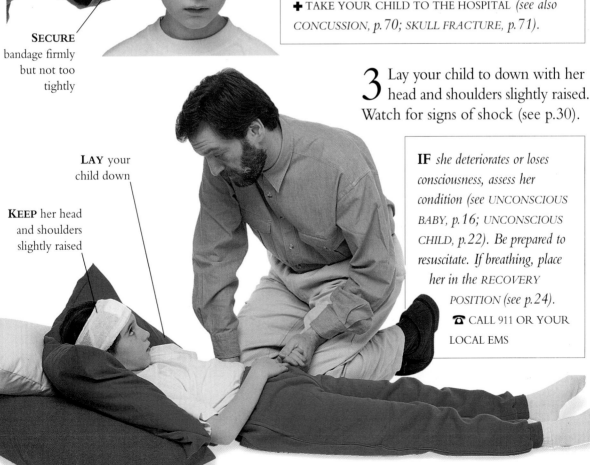

LAY your child down

KEEP her head and shoulders slightly raised

> **IF** *she deteriorates or loses consciousness, assess her condition (see* UNCONSCIOUS BABY, *p.16;* UNCONSCIOUS CHILD, *p.22). Be prepared to resuscitate. If breathing, place her in the* RECOVERY POSITION *(see p.24).*
> ☎ CALL 911 OR YOUR LOCAL EMS

CONCUSSION

The brain may be "shaken" by a violent blow, causing a concussion. The period of unconsciousness is usually brief and followed by complete recovery. You should be able to distinguish between a bump on the head with no concussion, a brief period of concussion (less than 20 seconds), and an extended period of unconsciousness.

Recognizing concussion • *Brief loss of consciousness, dizziness or nausea on recovery*
• *Loss of memory of immediately preceding events*
• *A mild headache.*

Conscious child

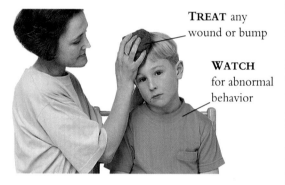

TREAT any wound or bump

WATCH for abnormal behavior

If your child has bumped his head, sit him down and treat any minor bruise or wound with a cold compress.

> **WATCH** *for signs of abnormal behavior. If he does not recover fully within a few minutes,* ℂ CALL A DOCTOR.

Child who regains consciousness quickly

1 If your child has been "knocked out," even briefly, ℂ CALL A DOCTOR.

2 Make her rest and watch her closely. If she does not recover completely within 30 minutes, ☎ CALL 911 OR YOUR LOCAL EMS.

WATCH child carefully for abnormal behavior

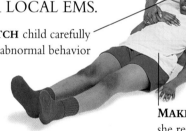

MAKE sure she rests

Unconscious child

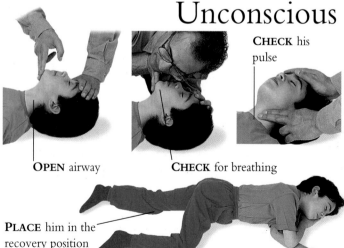

OPEN airway

CHECK his pulse

CHECK for breathing

PLACE him in the recovery position if breathing

☎ CALL 911 OR YOUR LOCAL EMS

Open his airway. Check his breathing and pulse (see UNCONSCIOUS BABY, p.16; UNCONSCIOUS CHILD, p.22). If breathing, place him in the RECOVERY POSITION (see p.24). Stay with him until the ambulance arrives.

SKULL FRACTURE

Fractures of the skull are potentially very serious injuries and require urgent medical attention to minimize the risk of damage to the brain and the possibility of infection.

Recognizing a skull fracture • *A wound or bruise on the head* • *A soft area on the scalp* • *Impaired consciousness* • *Deterioration in level of response* • *Clear or pinkish fluid or blood* *draining from the nose or ear(s)* • *Blood showing in the white of the eye* • *Distortion of the head or face.*

☎ CALL 911 OR YOUR LOCAL EMS

> **IF** *you suspect BACK OR NECK INJURIES, see pp. 73-75.* **DO NOT** *attempt to control fluids draining from the nose or ears.*

Unconscious child

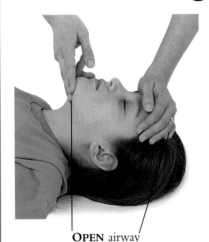

OPEN airway
(lift chin, DO NOT tilt head)

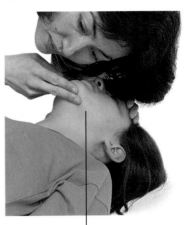

CHECK for breathing

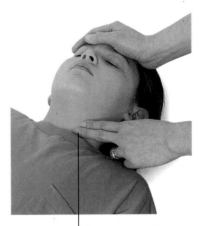

CHECK her pulse

1 Open your child's airway. Check her breathing and pulse (see UNCONSCIOUS BABY, p.16; UNCONSCIOUS CHILD, p.22).

2 Avoid any unnecesssary movement, since the skull fracture may be linked to a neck or spine injury. Stay with her and watch for any change in her condition while waiting for the ambulance to arrive.

Delayed reaction

There may be a serious reaction to a head injury hours or even days later. Cerebral compression is a condition caused by blood accumulating within the skull and putting pressure on the brain following a head injury.

Recognizing cerebral compression
• *Disorientation and confusion* • *A severe headache* • *Impaired consciousness* • *Noisy breathing, becoming slow* • *Slow but strong pulse* • *Unequal pupils* • *Weakness or paralysis* • *Elevated temperature* • *Seizure* • *Vomiting.* Be prepared to resuscitate (see UNCONSCIOUS BABY, p.16; UNCONSCIOUS CHILD, p.22).

☎ CALL 911 OR YOUR LOCAL EMS

BROKEN NOSE/CHEEKBONE

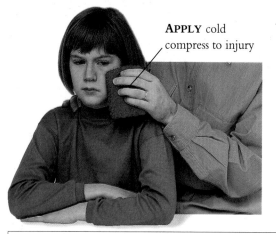

APPLY cold compress to injury

1 Sit your child down and apply a cold compress to the injured part. This helps reduce the swelling. Hold the compress in place for about 30 minutes.

2 If your child's nose is bleeding heavily, ask her to sit with her head over a bowl and to pinch her nostrils together.

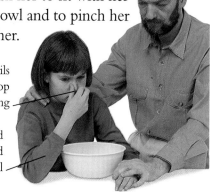

PINCH nostrils together to stop bleeding

SIT your child well forward over bowl

> **IF** *pinching her nose hurts too much, simply ask her to sit forward and give her a soft pad or towel to soak up the blood.*
> ✚ TAKE YOUR CHILD TO THE HOSPITAL

72

BROKEN JAW

Recognizing a broken jaw
• *Tender, swollen, bruised jaw* • *Teeth may be out of line.*

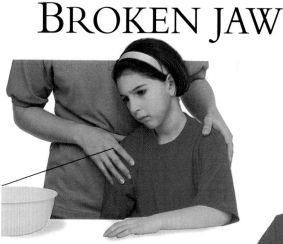

HELP her to lean forward

1 Sit her down with her head well forward. Tell her not to swallow, but to let any blood or saliva drain away.

HOLD pad against jaw and support jaw with your hand

> **IF** *she loses consciousness, assess her condition (see* UNCONSCIOUS BABY, *p.16;* UNCONSCIOUS CHILD, *p.22). Be prepared to resuscitate. If breathing, place in* RECOVERY POSITION *(p.24).*
> ☎ CALL 911 OR YOUR LOCAL EMS

2 Make a soft pad and hold it firmly under her injured jaw. Do not bandage the pad in place in case she vomits. Continue to support the jaw on the way to the hospital.

✚ TAKE YOUR CHILD TO THE HOSPITAL

BACK AND NECK INJURIES
The conscious child

☎ CALL 911 OR YOUR LOCAL EMS

DO NOT *move the injured child unless his life is in danger.* **IF** *you do have to move him, try to do so in "one piece," taking care not to twist or bend the neck or spine.*

REASSURE your child

HOLD his head in your hands

KEEP his back straight

1 Reassure your child and tell him not to move. Steady and support his head and neck by placing your hands over his ears and keeping his head in line with his spine. Be careful not to pull on his neck.

2 Keep his head supported in this position until help arrives. Ask someone to put rolled blankets or towels around his neck and shoulders for extra support.

MAINTAIN support of his head

PLACE rolled blankets around his head and shoulders

PLACE folded blankets or towels either side of his body

3 If assistance is delayed, get a helper to arrange rolled towels or blankets around your child's neck and shoulders and on either side of his body to stabilize his position while you continue to keep his head steady. Be careful not to move your child in the process.

CONTINUE to support his head

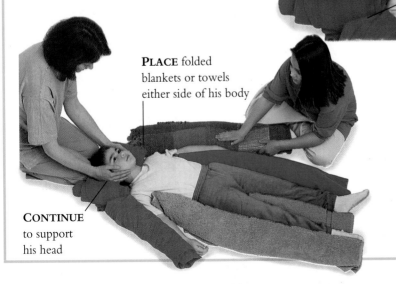

73

BACK AND NECK INJURIES
The unconscious child

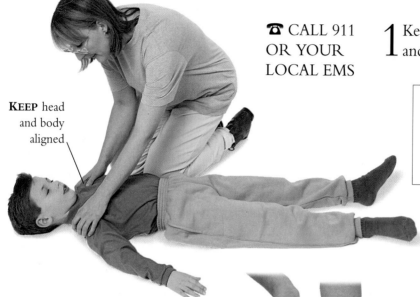

☎ CALL 911
OR YOUR
LOCAL EMS

KEEP head
and body
aligned

1 Keep your child's head, trunk and toes in a straight line.

DO NOT *move your child unless you think his life is in immediate danger. He is at risk of paralysis.*

OPEN airway

LIFT his chin

2 Place two fingers under the chin and lift the jaw very gently to open the airway. Do not tilt the head.

DO NOT tilt head

CONTINUE to support his head

CHECK for breathing

3 Check for breathing (see UNCONSCIOUS BABY, p.16; UNCONSCIOUS CHILD, p.22).

4 With the palm of your hand still supporting your child's head, check his pulse (see UNCONSCIOUS BABY, p.16; UNCONSCIOUS CHILD, p.22). Be prepared to resuscitate.

CHECK his pulse

CONTINUE to support his head

74

Rolling an unconscious child

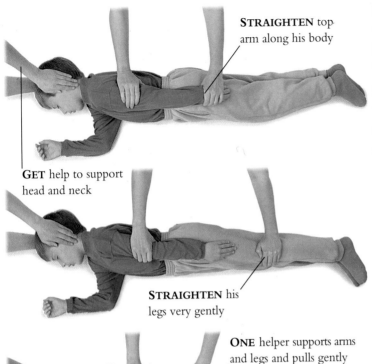

STRAIGHTEN top arm along his body

GET help to support head and neck

STRAIGHTEN his legs very gently

ONE helper supports arms and legs and pulls gently

KEEP head in line with body while he is turned

DO NOT tilt head

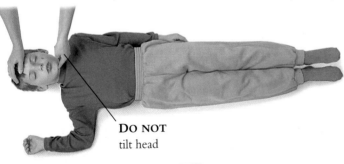

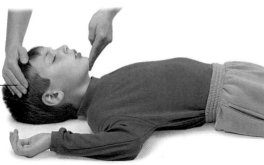

KEEP head and neck supported until ambulance arrives

If you need to resuscitate a child who has stopped breathing and is lying on his stomach or side, the "log-roll" technique must be used to turn him onto his back. It is vital to keep the child's head, body, and feet in a straight line. You will need a helper to do this safely.

1 While one adult holds the child's head, the other should gently straighten his top arm down his side.

2 Straighten his legs, so that they are in line with his back and head.

3 In one synchronized movement, roll the child onto his back by gently pulling at his arm and hips, keeping the head and body in a straight line throughout.

4 Lift his chin very slightly to open his airway. You can then resuscitate (see UNCONSCIOUS BABY, p.16; UNCONSCIOUS CHILD, p.22).

5 Keep him in this position, supporting his head continually, until the ambulance arrives. Treat for shock (see p.30).

75

BROKEN LEG

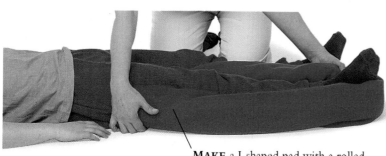

SUPPORT leg at joints above and below injury

MAKE a J-shaped pad with a rolled blanket and place it around his leg

1 Lay your child down gently and support his leg at the ankle and knee joints. If other adults are present, ask one to help you.

2 Steady the injured leg with padding. Place a rolled-up blanket, folded around the foot to extend up between the legs. If necessary, cover him with another blanket to keep him warm.

☎ CALL 911 OR YOUR LOCAL EMS

76

Making binder and cravat bandages

TAKE a triangular bandage

FOLD top point over to touch the base

BINDER BANDAGE

FOLD bandage in half to make a binder bandage

CRAVAT BANDAGE

FOLD bandage in half again to make a cravat bandage

Tying a square knot

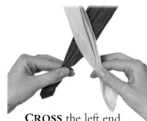

CROSS the left end (yellow) over the right (blue)

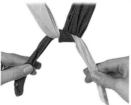

TAKE the yellow under and through

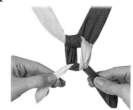

PASS the yellow over the blue and through the gap

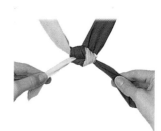

PULL the ends firmly

How to splint an injured leg

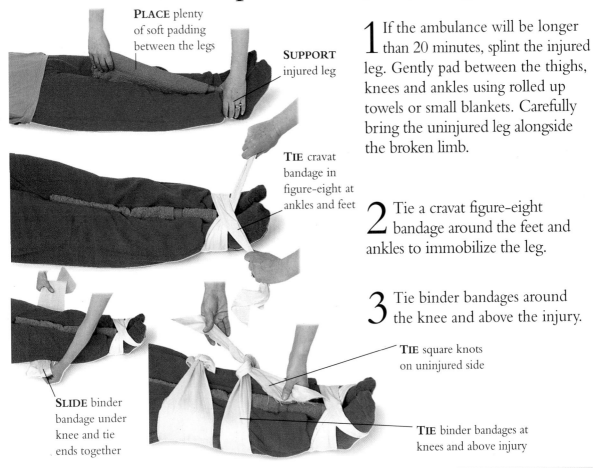

PLACE plenty of soft padding between the legs

SUPPORT injured leg

TIE cravat bandage in figure-eight at ankles and feet

SLIDE binder bandage under knee and tie ends together

1 If the ambulance will be longer than 20 minutes, splint the injured leg. Gently pad between the thighs, knees and ankles using rolled up towels or small blankets. Carefully bring the uninjured leg alongside the broken limb.

2 Tie a cravat figure-eight bandage around the feet and ankles to immobilize the leg.

3 Tie binder bandages around the knee and above the injury.

TIE square knots on uninjured side

TIE binder bandages at knees and above injury

77

BROKEN PELVIS

☎ CALL 911 OR YOUR LOCAL EMS

INJURIES *to the pelvis are usually caused by crushing or direct impact. There may be* INTERNAL BLEEDING *(p.57).* SHOCK *may develop (p.30).*

Recognizing a broken pelvis
• *Inability to walk or stand* • *Pain and tenderness in the hip and groin region* • *Bleeding from the urinary orifice.*

Lay your child down gently, keeping her head low. Calm her. Treat for shock, if necessary, by covering her with a blanket.

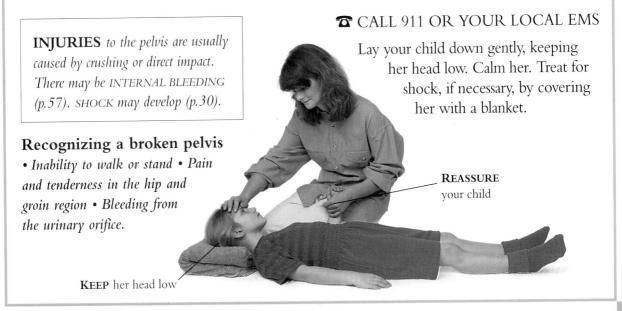

REASSURE your child

KEEP her head low

KNEE INJURY

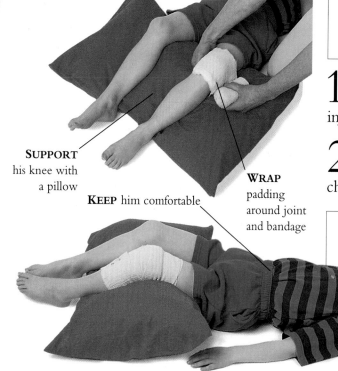

THIS *technique should be performed by the rescuer only if emergency medical services are unavailable or hours away.*

1 Help him lie down, then slide a pillow under the injured knee. Pad around the injured knee with cotton or a soft dressing.

2 Use a roller bandage to keep the padding in place, working from the child's injured side.

SUPPORT his knee with a pillow

WRAP padding around joint and bandage

KEEP him comfortable

DO NOT *attempt to force the knee straight since this may cause further injury.*

DO NOT *allow the child to eat, drink, or walk.*

☎ CALL 911 OR YOUR LOCAL EMS

BROKEN FOOT

Fractures of the foot are usually caused by crushing.

Recognizing a broken foot
• *Bruising and swelling* • *Stiffness*
• *Difficulty in walking.*

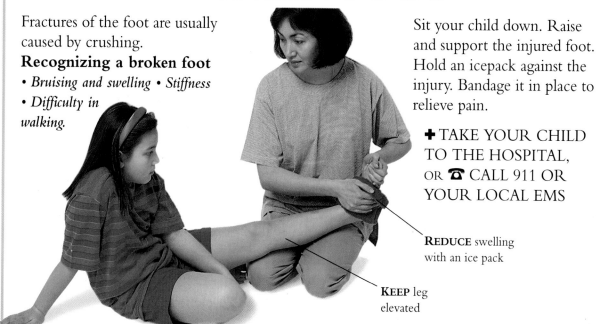

Sit your child down. Raise and support the injured foot. Hold an icepack against the injury. Bandage it in place to relieve pain.

✚ TAKE YOUR CHILD TO THE HOSPITAL, OR ☎ CALL 911 OR YOUR LOCAL EMS

REDUCE swelling with an ice pack

KEEP leg elevated

78

BROKEN COLLAR BONE

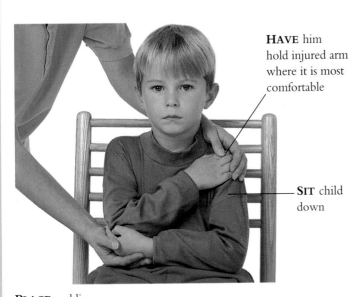

HAVE him hold injured arm where it is most comfortable

SIT child down

The collar bone may be broken by indirect force if a child falls onto his outstretched hand, or by a blow to his shoulder.

Recognizing a broken collar bone • *Pain and tenderness increased by movement* • *Head turned and inclined to the injured side.*

1 Sit your child down while he holds his injured arm across his chest. Ask him to support his elbow in his other hand.

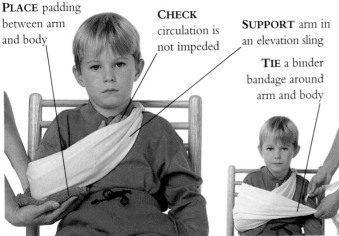

PLACE padding between arm and body

CHECK circulation is not impeded

SUPPORT arm in an elevation sling

TIE a binder bandage around arm and body

2 Place your child's arm in an ELEVATION SLING for support (see p.111).

3 Secure the arm with a BINDER BANDAGE (see p.76 and below). Check his fingers frequently for color, temperature, or numbness.
✚ TAKE YOUR CHILD TO THE HOSPITAL, OR
☎ CALL 911 OR YOUR LOCAL EMS

Tying a binder bandage around a sling

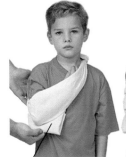

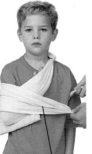

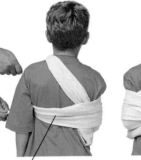

A sling will support an injured arm, but a binder bandage provides extra support and prevents movement when you take your child to the hospital.

SLIDE padding between arm and body

PLACE a binder bandage around body and arm

SECURE with a square knot tied on uninjured side

BROKEN ARM

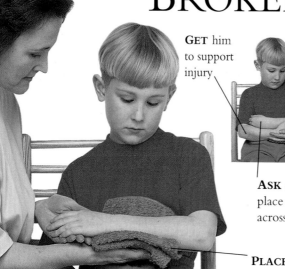

GET him to support injury

ASK child to place his arm across chest

PLACE padding around injury

The treatment described below is suitable for injuries to the upper arm, forearm, and wrist.

1 Sit your child down and if possible get him to support his injured arm in his hand.

2 Place a pad between his arm and his chest to immobilize and cushion the injured limb.

3 Put the injured limb in an ARM SLING (see p.110), secured with a SQUARE KNOT (see p.76).

4 For additional support, place a BINDER BANDAGE over the sling and around your child's arm and chest (see p.76 and p.79).

✚ TAKE YOUR CHILD TO THE HOSPITAL

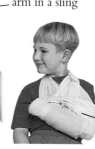

SUPPORT arm in a sling

TIE a binder bandage around arm and chest

80

BROKEN ELBOW

LAY child down

HAVE child place injured arm across his body

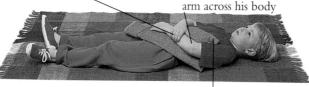

PUT soft padding between his arm and body

Elbow injuries need special care and prompt treatment in the hospital. **Recognizing a broken elbow** • *Pain increased by attempted movement* • *Stiffness* • *Swelling or bruising.*

BANDAGE upper arm to chest with binder bandage

DO NOT *attempt to straighten or bend the elbow. Make sure the bandages are not too tight.*

☎ CALL 911 OR YOUR LOCAL EMS

SECURE wrist and lower arm to hips with binder bandage

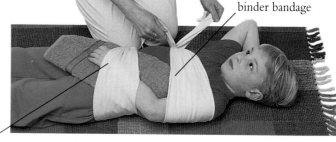

BROKEN RIBS

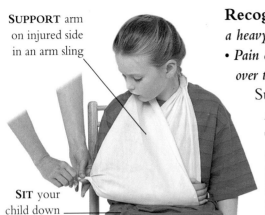

SUPPORT arm on injured side in an arm sling

SIT your child down

Recognizing broken ribs • *Child has had a blow to chest, a heavy fall, or has been crushed* • *Sharp pain at the fracture site* • *Pain on breathing* • *Signs of internal bleeding* • *Open wound over the fracture site.*

Support the arm on the injured side in an ARM SLING (see p.110).

✚ TAKE YOUR CHILD TO THE HOSPITAL, OR ☎ CALL 911 OR YOUR LOCAL EMS

IF *she has a CHEST WOUND (see p.58) or INTERNAL BLEEDING (see p.57),* ☎ CALL 911 OR YOUR LOCAL EMS.

Open or multiple rib fractures

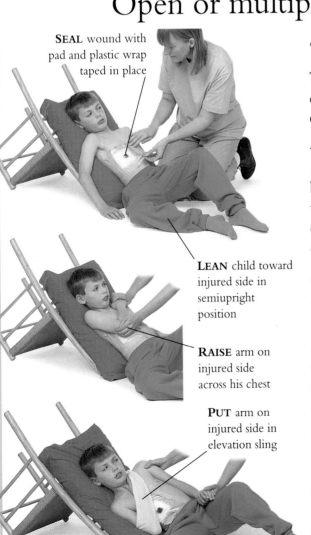

SEAL wound with pad and plastic wrap taped in place

LEAN child toward injured side in semiupright position

RAISE arm on injured side across his chest

PUT arm on injured side in elevation sling

☎ CALL 911 OR YOUR LOCAL EMS

Treat any open wound and support the chest wall to safeguard breathing (see also CHEST WOUND, p.58).

1 Help your child into a semiupright position supported by pillows. Incline his body toward the injured side. Cover any wounds to the chest wall using a sterile dressing sealed with plastic wrap, leaving one corner untaped to permit exhaled air to escape.

2 Place the arm on the injured side across your child's chest.

3 Use an ELEVATION SLING (see p.111) to support the raised arm. Keep him as comfortable as possible while you wait for the ambulance. Check fingers frequently for color, temperature, or numbness.

IF *your child loses consciousness or develops breathing difficulties, assess his condition (see UNCONSCIOUS BABY, p.16; UNCONSCIOUS CHILD, p.22). Be prepared to resuscitate.*

81

BROKEN HAND

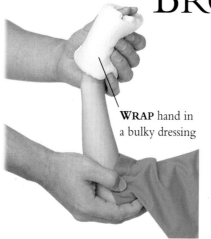

1 Wrap the injured hand in a bulky dressing. Raise your child's hand, supporting it to minimize swelling.

WRAP hand in a bulky dressing

IF *there is a wound, control the bleeding by raising the hand and applying gentle pressure over a clean dressing.*

COVER any wound with a dressing

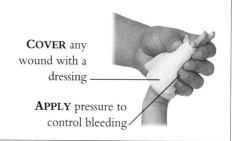

APPLY pressure to control bleeding

2 Place arm in an ELEVATION SLING (see p.111) to reduce swelling and prevent movement of the injured hand. Check fingers for color, temperature, or numbness.

SUPPORT hand and arm in elevation sling

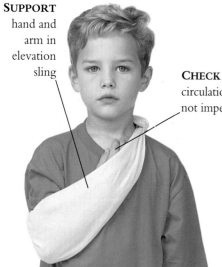

CHECK circulation is not impeded

TIE binder bandage around arm and body

3 Tie a BINDER BANDAGE (see pp.76 and 79) around the arm, securing it with a knot tied on the uninjured side.
✚ TAKE YOUR CHILD TO THE HOSPITAL

82

TRAPPED FINGERS

COOL injury by holding her fingers under running water

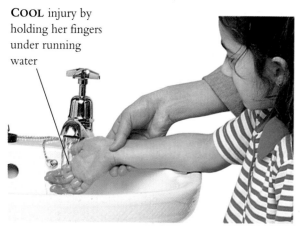

After the trapped fingers are released, hold them under cool running water for a few minutes to relieve the pain and minimize swelling. If the fingers still hurt, apply a COLD COMPRESS (see p.84).

IF *after half an hour the fingers are still swollen and movement is impaired, they may be broken.*
✚ TAKE YOUR CHILD TO THE HOSPITAL

SPRAINED ANKLE

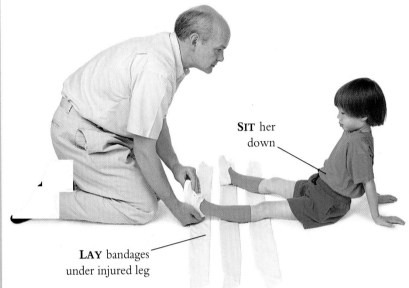

SIT her down

LAY bandages under injured leg

Suspect an ankle sprain if your child can't take her full weight on her foot after she falls or twists her ankle.

1 Sit your child down to rest her foot. Leave her shoe on. Place two or three binder bandages under the injured leg, supporting the ankle as you do so.

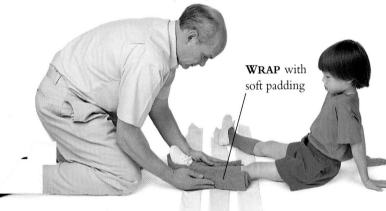

WRAP with soft padding

2 Wrap the foot, ankle, and lower leg in a thick layer of soft padding, so that the joint is supported above and below the ankle.

83

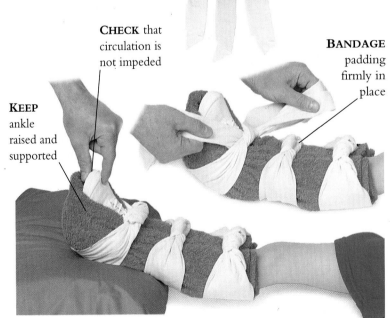

CHECK that circulation is not impeded

BANDAGE padding firmly in place

KEEP ankle raised and supported

3 Bandage the padding firmly in place with the binder bandages, ensuring that the bandage nearest the ankle is around the heel also.

4 Raise and support the foot to minimize swelling and check circulation.

✆ CALL A DOCTOR
OR
✚ TAKE YOUR CHILD TO THE HOSPITAL

BRUISES AND SWELLINGS

After a fall or bump, bruising and swelling may develop rapidly. Resting, cooling, applying direct pressure, and elevating the injury will alleviate symptoms.

1 Make your child comfortable. Raise and support the injury to rest it.

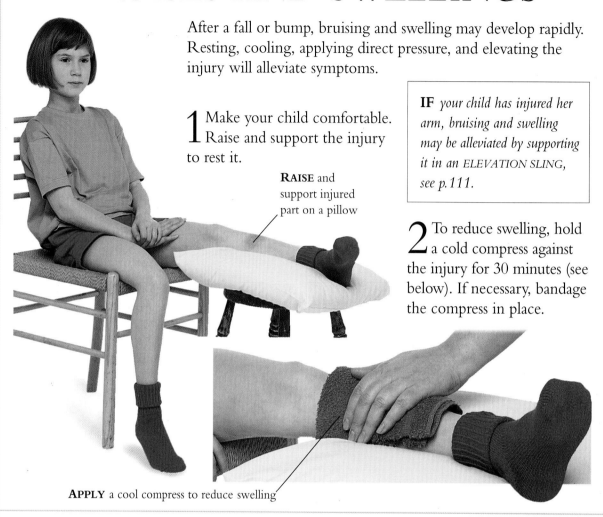

RAISE and support injured part on a pillow

IF *your child has injured her arm, bruising and swelling may be alleviated by supporting it in an ELEVATION SLING, see p.111.*

2 To reduce swelling, hold a cold compress against the injury for 30 minutes (see below). If necessary, bandage the compress in place.

APPLY a cool compress to reduce swelling

84

Making a cold compress

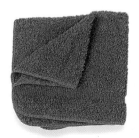

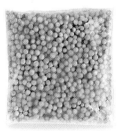

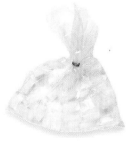

A cold compress minimizes swelling and pain by reducing blood flow to the injured area. Leave a compress on the injury for about 30 minutes, changing it when necessary. If possible, the compress should be left uncovered, but if you need to secure it in place, use a gauze bandage or other open-weave material.

Cloth: wring it out in cold water and replace every ten minutes.

Bag of frozen peas: wrap in a light towel before placing it on the injury.

Ice: fill a plastic bag two-thirds full of ice and add a little salt to help the ice melt, then seal.

SPLINTER

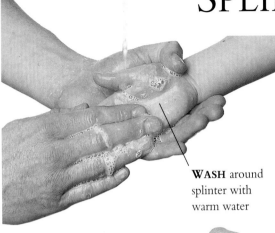

WASH around splinter with warm water

1 Clean the area around the splinter with soap and warm water.

> **IF** *your child is not inoculated against* TETANUS *(p.50),* © CALL A DOCTOR.

> **DO NOT** *poke at the area with a needle.*

2 Sterilize a pair of tweezers by passing them through a flame. Allow the tweezers to cool. Don't touch the ends or wipe off the soot.

STERILIZE tweezers in a flame

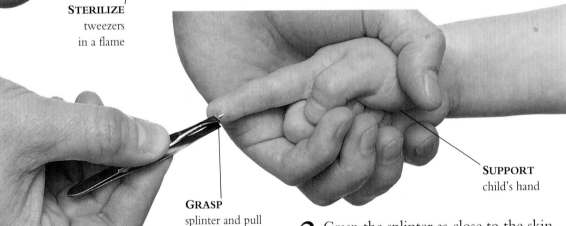

SUPPORT child's hand

GRASP splinter and pull straight out

3 Grasp the splinter as close to the skin as possible, and draw it back out at the angle it went in.

> **IF** *the splinter doesn't come out easily, or if it breaks,* © CALL A DOCTOR.

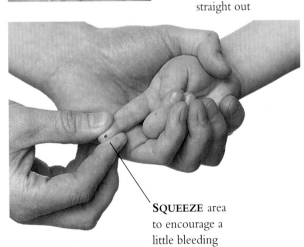

SQUEEZE area to encourage a little bleeding

4 Squeeze the wound to encourage a little bleeding that will flush out dirt. Wash the area again, pat it dry thoroughly, and cover with an adhesive bandage.

EYE

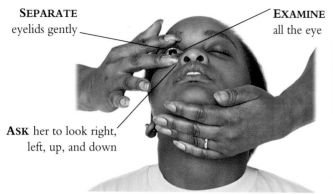

SEPARATE eyelids gently

EXAMINE all the eye

ASK her to look right, left, up, and down

> **DO NOT** *touch, or attempt to remove, any foreign body that is sticking to, or embedded in, the eye (see below).*

1 Sit your child down, facing the light. Separate the eyelids. Ask her to look right, left, up, and down. Examine all of the eye.

TRY to wash out foreign body

LIFT off foreign body with a damp handkerchief

USE a bowl to catch water

2 If you can see the foreign body, wash it out using a jug of clean water. Tilt her head and aim for the inner corner so that water will wash over the eye, or use the corner of a damp handkerchief to lift it off.

3 If an object is under the eyelid, you can ask an older child to clear it herself by lifting the upper eyelid over the lower. You will need to do this for a younger child; wrap her in a towel first to keep her from grabbing your arms.

LIFT upper eyelid over lower lid

IF *eye is still red or sore,*
✚ TAKE HER TO THE HOSPITAL.

A foreign body that cannot be removed

Cover the eye with a pad and bandage so that a gentle pressure is exerted. Then bandage both eyes, to keep blood, fluid, and dirt out of the uninjured eye. Reassure her.

✚ TAKE HER TO THE HOSPITAL

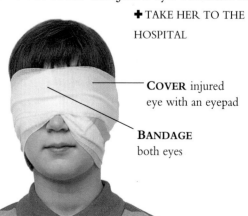

COVER injured eye with an eyepad

BANDAGE both eyes

86

EAR

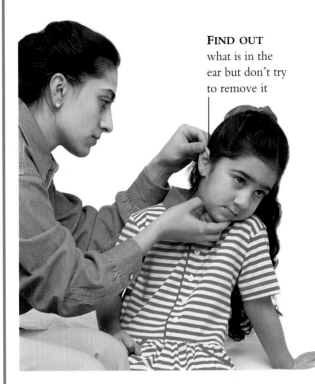

FIND OUT what is in the ear but don't try to remove it

Children often push things into their ears. A hard object may become stuck, causing pain and temporary deafness; it may damage the ear drum.

> **DO NOT** *attempt to remove the object.*

Reassure your child and ask her what she put into her ear. Don't try to remove the object, even if you can see it.

✚ TAKE YOUR CHILD TO THE HOSPITAL

87

An insect in the ear

If an insect flies or crawls into her ear your child may be very alarmed. Sit her down and support her head with the affected ear uppermost. Gently flood the ear with tepid water so that the insect floats out.

> **IF** *you can't remove the insect,*
> **✚ TAKE YOUR CHILD TO THE HOSPITAL.**

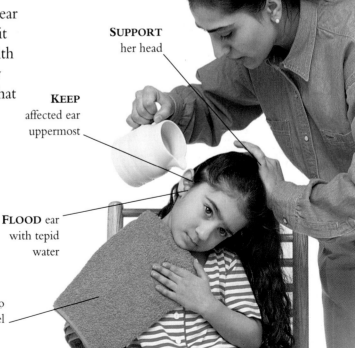

SUPPORT her head

KEEP affected ear uppermost

FLOOD ear with tepid water

ASK her to hold a towel

NOSE

Recognizing foreign body in the nose
• *Difficult or noisy breathing through nose* • *Swelling of nose* • *Smelly or blood-stained discharge indicates object has been present for a while.*

Calm and reassure your child and tell him to breathe through his mouth.

KEEP him calm

ASK him to breathe through his mouth

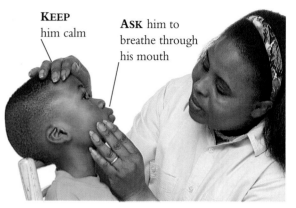

DO NOT *attempt to remove the object.*
✚ TAKE YOUR CHILD TO THE HOSPITAL

SWALLOWED OBJECT

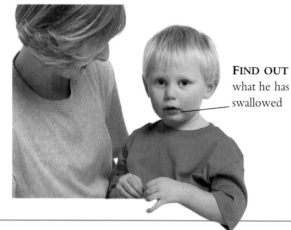

FIND OUT what he has swallowed

Find out what your child has swallowed. If the object is small and smooth like a pebble or a coin, there is little danger.

℃ CALL A DOCTOR

IF *the object is sharp or large, don't give your child anything to eat or drink.*
✚ TAKE YOUR CHILD TO THE HOSPITAL

INHALED FOREIGN BODY

Small, smooth objects can slip into the airway. Nuts are a danger in children since they can be inhaled into the lungs.

Encourage your child to cough. If she can't cough, breathe, or speak, give her abdominal thrusts if she is a child, or back blows and chest thrusts if she is an infant. If she continues to choke, see CHOKING BABY, p.36; CHOKING CHILD, p.38.

℃ CALL A DOCTOR OR
✚ TAKE HER TO THE HOSPITAL

STAND behind her and wrap your arms around her waist

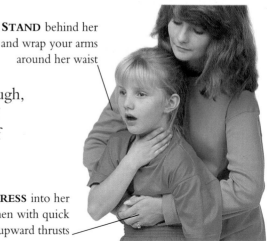

PRESS into her abdomen with quick upward thrusts

ANIMAL BITE
Superficial bite

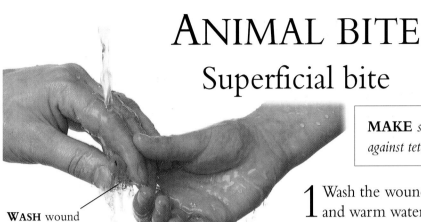

WASH wound with soap and warm, running water

DRY wound and cover with an adhesive bandage

> **MAKE** *sure your child is protected against tetanus infection (see p.50).*

1 Wash the wound thoroughly, using soap and warm water. Rinse the wound under running water for at least five minutes to wash away any dirt.

2 Gently, but thoroughly, pat the wound dry with a clean pad or tissue. Cover it with an adhesive bandage or a small sterile dressing.

✚ TAKE YOUR CHILD TO THE HOSPITAL

Serious bite

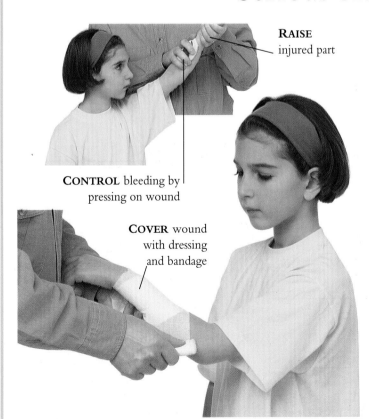

RAISE injured part

CONTROL bleeding by pressing on wound

COVER wound with dressing and bandage

1 Apply direct pressure over the wound, preferably over a clean dressing or pad. Lift and support the injured part above the level of your child's heart.

> **IF** *the bleeding is severe, see* BLEEDING, *p.46.*

2 Cover the wound with a sterile dressing and bandage firmly in place.

✚ TAKE YOUR CHILD TO THE HOSPITAL

> **IF** *your child is bitten by an animal that is behaving strangely or foaming at the mouth, take her to the hospital for antirabies injections. If possible, trap the animal so it can be tested for rabies.*

INSECT STING

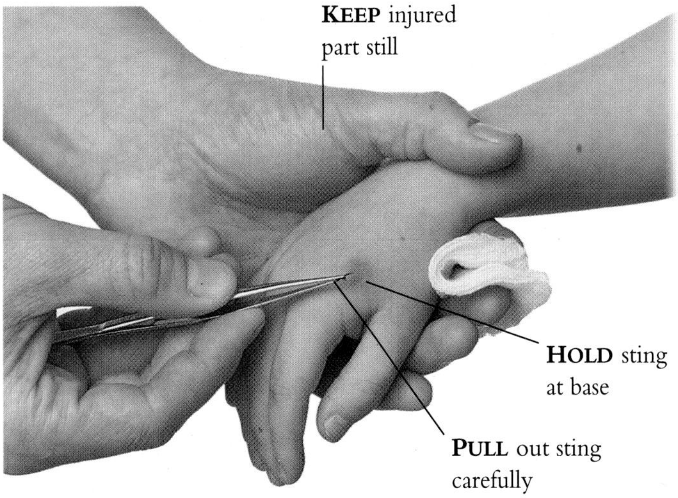
KEEP injured part still
HOLD sting at base
PULL out sting carefully

1 If the sting is still in the skin, remove it with tweezers or scrape it off with a credit card. Grasp the sting as close to the skin as possible and carefully pull it out. Don't grasp the sting at the top. You may squeeze the poison sac and the poison will enter the wound.

> **IF** *your child collapses, she may be allergic to the sting. Treat as for* ANAPHYLACTIC SHOCK, *opposite.*

Sting in mouth

To reduce swelling, give your child an ice cube to suck or cold water to drink.

✆ CALL A DOCTOR

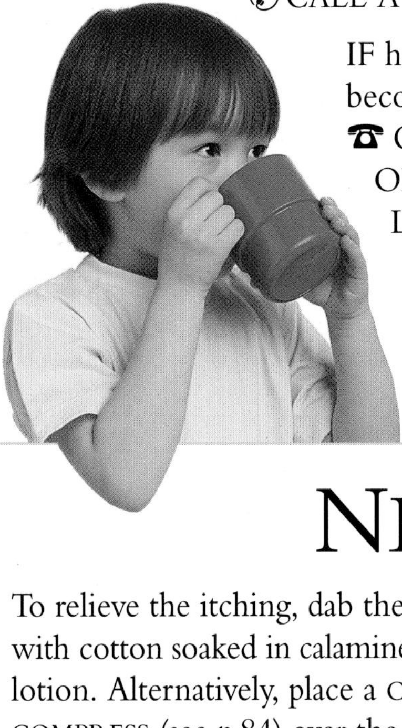

IF her breathing becomes difficult,
☎ CALL 911 OR YOUR LOCAL EMS.

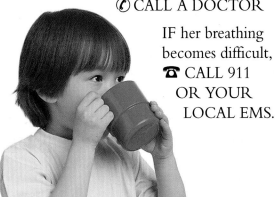

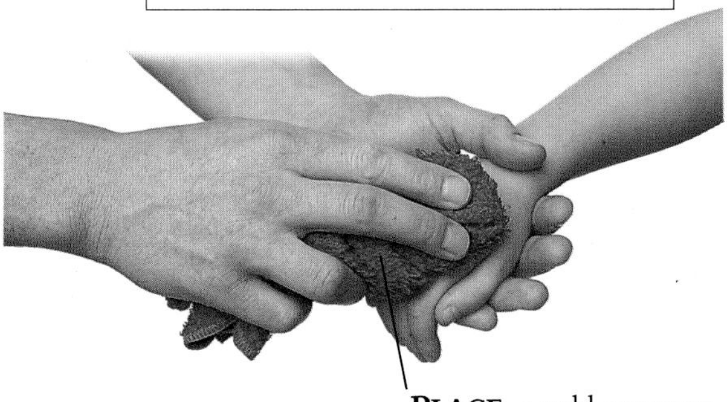
PLACE a cold compress over injury

2 Cool the area with a COLD COMPRESS (see p.84) to minimize the pain and swelling. Leave the compress in place until the pain is relieved, about ten minutes. Rest the injured part.

NETTLE RASH

To relieve the itching, dab the rash with cotton soaked in calamine lotion. Alternatively, place a COLD COMPRESS (see p.84) over the rash until the pain is relieved, about ten minutes. If the rash is extensive, ✆ CALL A DOCTOR.

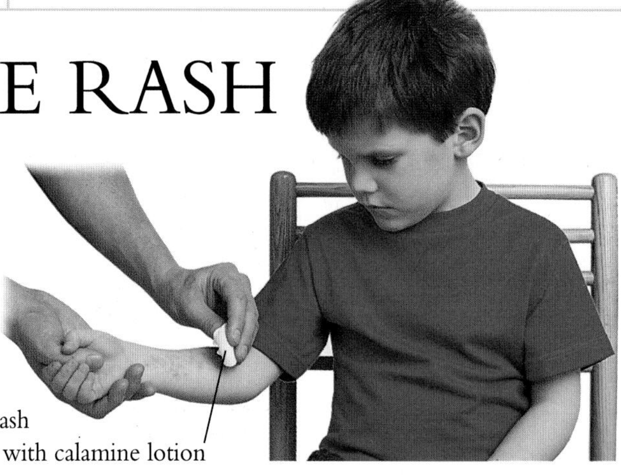
SOOTHE rash by dabbing with calamine lotion

ANAPHYLACTIC SHOCK

This is a severe, life-threatening allergic reaction that may develop within a few minutes following the injection of a particular drug, the sting of an insect or marine creature, or the ingestion of a particular food.

The reaction causes constriction of the air passages. Swelling of the face and neck increases the risk of suffocation.

Recognizing anaphylactic shock
• *Anxiety* • *Red, blotchy skin* • *Swelling of the face and neck* • *Puffiness around the eyes* • *Hives* • *Wheezing* • *Difficult breathing* • *Rapid pulse.*

☎ CALL 911 OR YOUR LOCAL EMS

IF *your child loses consciousness, assess his condition (see UNCONSCIOUS BABY, p.16; UNCONSCIOUS CHILD, p.22). If breathing, place him in the RECOVERY POSITION (see p.24). Be prepared to resuscitate.*

A CHILD *with a known allergy may have medication, often called a "sting kit," to take in case of an attack. Use this medication as soon as the attack starts. Follow the directions carefully.*

Help your child into the position that most relieves his breathing difficulty. Talk to him calmly and reassure him while you wait for the ambulance to arrive.

SUPPORT him in a position that helps his breathing

LOOSEN tight clothing at neck and waist

MARINE STINGS
Jellyfish sting

Jellyfish venom is contained in stinging cells that stick to a child's skin. The sting is painful, but usually not serious. A similar reaction is produced by sea anemones and corals.

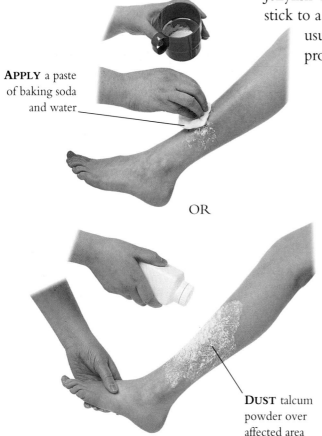

APPLY a paste of baking soda and water

OR

IF *your child develops a severe allergic reaction, see ANAPHYLACTIC SHOCK, p.91.* ☎ CALL 911 OR YOUR LOCAL EMS

Make a paste of baking soda and water and apply it to the wound.

OR

Dust a dry powder, such as talcum powder or meat tenderizer, over the skin around the injury.

DUST talcum powder over affected area

IF *the skin is very red and painful,*
✚TAKE YOUR CHILD TO THE HOSPITAL.

Weever fish sting

When trodden on, the spines from weever fish can puncture the skin, causing painful swelling and soreness. The spines may break off and become embedded in the foot.

Immerse the injury in water as hot as your child can bear for at least 30 minutes. Add more hot water as the water cools but be careful not to scald her.

IF *any spines remain, or the foot starts to swell,*
✚TAKE YOUR CHILD TO THE HOSPITAL.

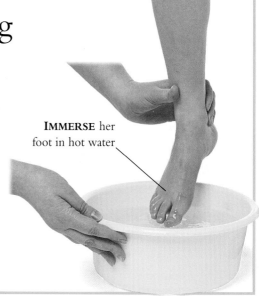

IMMERSE her foot in hot water

SNAKE BITE

Recognizing a snake bite
- *A pair of puncture marks*
- *Severe pain, redness, and swelling around bite* • *Vomiting* • *Disturbed vision* • *Breathing difficulties*
- *Increased salivation and sweating.*

IF *your child develops* ANAPHYLACTIC SHOCK, *see p.91.* **IF** *she loses consciousness, see* UNCONSCIOUS BABY, *p.16;* UNCONSCIOUS CHILD, *p.22. Be prepared to resuscitate. If breathing, place her in the* RECOVERY POSITION *(see p.24).*

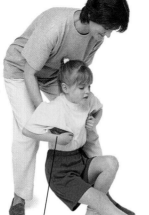

HELP her to sit down

1 Help your child to sit or lie down, making sure that the wounded part is *below* the level of her heart.

DO NOT *let your child walk.*
DO NOT *apply a tourniquet, or cut the wound, or try to suck out the venom. An accurate description of the snake will help doctors treat the injury.*

KEEP injury below level of heart

2 Reassure her. Keep her calm and still to keep the venom from spreading through her body. Wash the wound gently with soap and water if available.

93

REASSURE child and keep her still

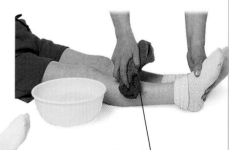

WASH wound gently with soap and water

3 Immobilize the injured area using padding and binder and cravat bandages at knees and ankles (see p.76).

☎ CALL 911 OR YOUR LOCAL EMS OR
✚ TAKE YOUR CHILD TO THE HOSPITAL IMMEDIATELY

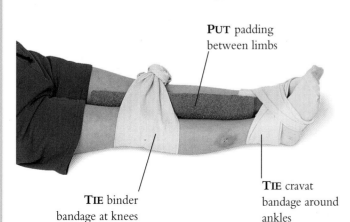

PUT padding between limbs

TIE binder bandage at knees

TIE cravat bandage around ankles

HYPOTHERMIA

Hypothermia occurs when the body temperature falls, and is extremely dangerous. An older child is most likely to develop hypothermia after over-exertion outside in poor weather conditions, or after falling into very cold water. For babies, see opposite.

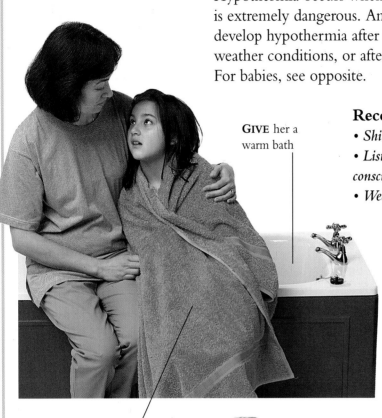

GIVE her a warm bath

Recognizing hypothermia
- *Shivering* • *Cold, pale, dry skin*
- *Listlessness or confusion* • *Failing consciousness* • *Slow, shallow breathing*
- *Weakening pulse.*

☎ CALL 911 OR YOUR LOCAL EMS

1 Give your child a warm bath, if she is able to climb in herself. When her skin color has returned to normal, help her out, dry her quickly, and wrap her in warm towels or blankets.

WRAP her in warm towels

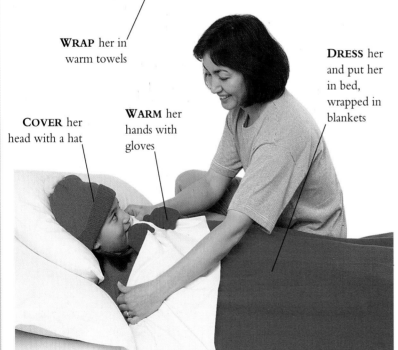

COVER her head with a hat

WARM her hands with gloves

DRESS her and put her in bed, wrapped in blankets

2 Dress your child with warm clothes and put her in bed, covered with plenty of blankets. Cover her head with a hat and make sure that the room is warm. Stay with her.

> **DO NOT** *put a source of direct heat, such as a hot-water bottle, next to the child's skin. The child must warm up gradually.*

94

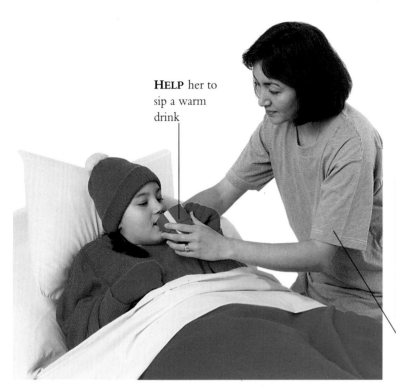

HELP her to sip a warm drink

3 If she is conscious, give your child a warm drink and some high-energy foods, such as chocolate. Do not leave her alone until you are sure that her color and temperature have returned to normal.

> **IF** *your child loses consciousness, assess her condition (see* UNCONSCIOUS BABY, p.16; UNCONSCIOUS CHILD, p.22). *Be prepared to resuscitate.*
> ☎ CALL 911 OR YOUR LOCAL EMS

STAY with her until color and temperature have returned to normal

95

Hypothermia in babies

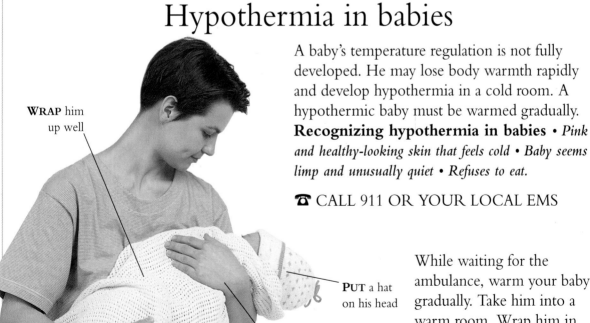

WRAP him up well

A baby's temperature regulation is not fully developed. He may lose body warmth rapidly and develop hypothermia in a cold room. A hypothermic baby must be warmed gradually.
Recognizing hypothermia in babies • *Pink and healthy-looking skin that feels cold • Baby seems limp and unusually quiet • Refuses to eat.*

☎ CALL 911 OR YOUR LOCAL EMS

PUT a hat on his head

While waiting for the ambulance, warm your baby gradually. Take him into a warm room. Wrap him in blankets. Put a hat on his head and cuddle him against your body so that he is warmed by your body heat.

CUDDLE him against your body

FROSTBITE

REMOVE clothing from affected area carefully

If children are accidentally exposed to extremely cold weather conditions, the tissues of the fingers and toes may freeze. Get your child to shelter before you start treatment. **Recognizing frostbite** • *Affected area feels like pins and needles* • *Numbness* • *Skin feeling hard and stiff, turning white and waxy.*

1 Take your child into a warm place. Sit her down, then very gently remove her socks and shoes.

TAKE her gloves off very carefully

2 Remove gloves and any rings. Undo her coat. Tell her to warm her hands under her armpits.

WARM hands with her own body heat, under armpits

3 When feet or toes are frostbitten, warm them gently by soaking them in warm (not hot) water. Do not allow the frostbitten area to touch the container.

THAW feet in warm water

DO NOT *warm by rubbing or with direct heat, such as hot-water bottles.* **NEVER** *burst blisters.*

COVER with light dressing and bandage if color does not return

4 If the skin is broken or the color does not return rapidly, apply a soft gauze dressing and bandage it lightly in place.
✚ TAKE YOUR CHILD TO THE HOSPITAL

HEAT EXHAUSTION

This condition may develop in hot, humid weather and is caused by dehydration. Children who are sick, particularly with diarrhea and vomiting, and those not used to playing in the heat are most at risk.

Recognizing heat exhaustion • *Headache and dizziness* • *Nausea* • *Sweating* • *Pale, clammy skin* • *Cramps* • *Rapid, weakening pulse.*

1 Take your child into the shade or into a cool room. Help him to lie down.

LAY child down in cool room

PUT folded towel or cushion under his head

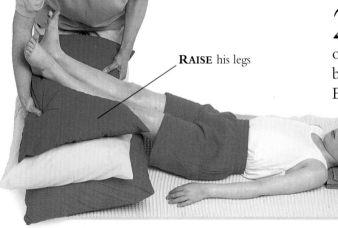

RAISE his legs

2 Raise and support your child's legs 8 to 12 inches on some pillows. This improves blood supply to the brain. Encourage him to rest.

97

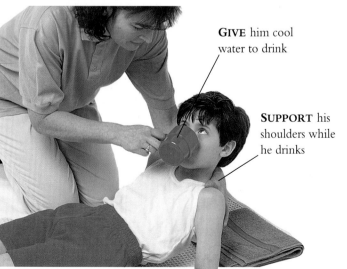

GIVE him cool water to drink

SUPPORT his shoulders while he drinks

3 Help your child to sit up and sip as much cool water or juice as he can manage.

IF *he loses consciousness, assess his condition (see* UNCONSCIOUS BABY, *p16;* UNCONSCIOUS CHILD, *p.22). Be prepared to resuscitate. If breathing, place him in the* RECOVERY POSITION *(see p.24).*

☎ CALL 911 OR YOUR LOCAL EMS

HEATSTROKE

If the body becomes severely overheated in hot surroundings, heatstroke may occur. It is a life-threatening emergency.

Recognizing heatstroke
• *Sudden onset of headache*
• *Confusion* • *Hot, flushed, dry skin* • *Rapid deterioration in level of response* • *Full, bounding pulse* • *Temperature above 104°F (40°C).*

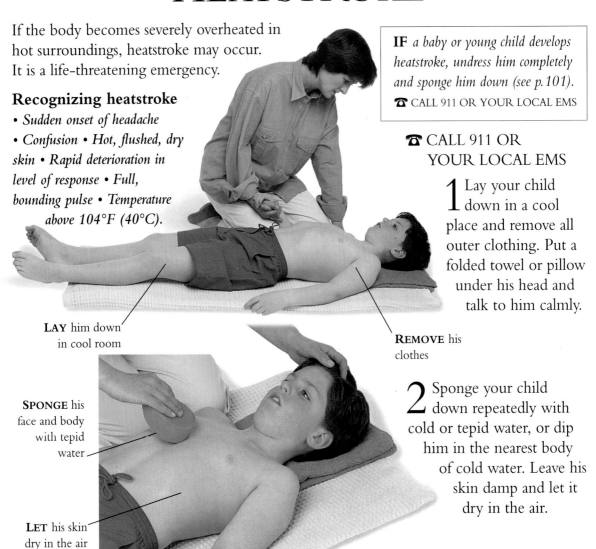

IF *a baby or young child develops heatstroke, undress him completely and sponge him down (see p.101).*
☎ CALL 911 OR YOUR LOCAL EMS

☎ CALL 911 OR YOUR LOCAL EMS

1 Lay your child down in a cool place and remove all outer clothing. Put a folded towel or pillow under his head and talk to him calmly.

LAY him down in cool room

REMOVE his clothes

SPONGE his face and body with tepid water

2 Sponge your child down repeatedly with cold or tepid water, or dip him in the nearest body of cold water. Leave his skin damp and let it dry in the air.

LET his skin dry in the air

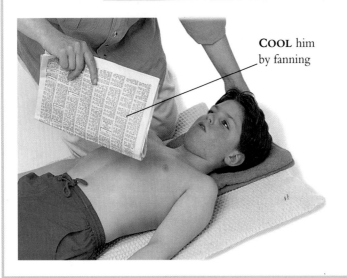

COOL him by fanning

3 Fan your child by hand or with an electric fan to bring his temperature down.

IF *he loses consciousness, assess his condition (see UNCONSCIOUS BABY, p.16; UNCONSCIOUS CHILD, p.22). Be prepared to resuscitate. If breathing, place him in the RECOVERY POSITION (see p.24).*
☎ CALL 911 OR YOUR LOCAL EMS

98

SUNBURN

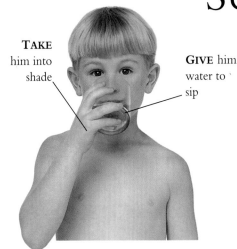

TAKE him into shade

GIVE him water to sip

Sunburned skin is red, itchy, and tender. Babies and young children are most vulnerable and should wear a hat and protective cream or clothing in the sun.

> **IF** *there is blistering,*
> ℂ CALL A DOCTOR.

1 Move your child into the shade or into a cool room and give him a cold drink.

2 Apply calamine lotion or a special after-sun cream to soothe the skin.

> **IF** *your child is restless, flushed, dizzy, has a temperature or headache, see HEATSTROKE, opposite.*

APPLY cooling cream to reduce discomfort

99

HEAT RASH

Recognizing heat rash • *A prickly, red rash particularly around the sweat glands on the chest and back and under the arms*

Sit your child down in a cool room and undress her. Sponge her down with cool water. Pat her almost dry with a soft towel, leaving the skin slightly damp. Apply calamine cream.

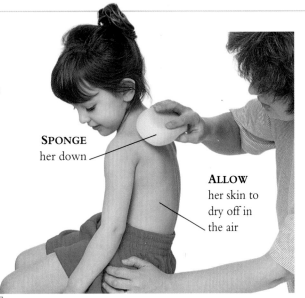

SPONGE her down

ALLOW her skin to dry off in the air

> **IF** *your baby develops heat rash, remove some of her clothes to cool her, or bathe her in tepid water. Dry her gently, leaving her skin slightly damp.*

> **IF** *the rash resembles blood under the skin,*
> ☎ CALL 911 OR YOUR LOCAL EMS.

FEVER

A body temperature that is above the normal level of 98.6°F (37°C) indicates a fever. An infection is the usual cause. If your child also has a bad headache, you should study the information on MENINGITIS (see opposite). A moderate fever is not harmful, but a temperature of above 104°F (40°C) can indicate serious illness, particularly in babies and very young children.

Recognizing a fever • *Raised temperature* • *A very pale face and a chilled feeling, with goose pimples* • *Shivering, with chattering teeth* As the fever advances • *Hot, flushed skin* • *General achiness* • *Sweating* • *Headache.*

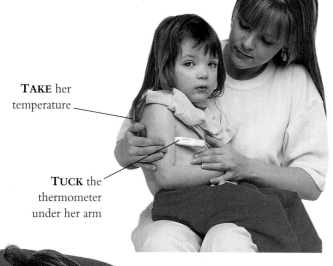

TAKE her temperature

TUCK the thermometer under her arm

1 Lift your child's arm and tuck the pointed end of the thermometer into her armpit. Fold her arm over her chest and leave the thermometer in place for the recommended time. A digital thermometer is the easiest to use.

LAY her down in bed or on the sofa

2 Make your child comfortable on a bed or sofa, but do not cover her. To help bring down her temperature, make sure she has plenty of water or diluted fruit juice to drink.

PROVIDE her with plenty to drink

GIVE her recommended dose of liquid acetaminophen

3 You can give your child the recommended dose of liquid acetaminophen to help reduce her temperature. If your child is very hot, sponge her down as well, (see opposite).

> **IF** *your baby is under three months old, she should not be given liquid acetaminophen, unless you are advised to do so by your doctor.*

100

Cooling babies and young children

In babies and children under four years of age, there is some risk of FEVER CONVULSIONS (see p.32). If your child's temperature rises above 104°F (40°C), ✆ CALL A DOCTOR.

Babies

Undress your baby down to his diaper and cool him by lightly sponging his body with tepid water. Try to keep him calm.

Young children

Undress your child and cool her by sponging her with tepid water. Continue for up to 30 minutes. Take her temperature again.

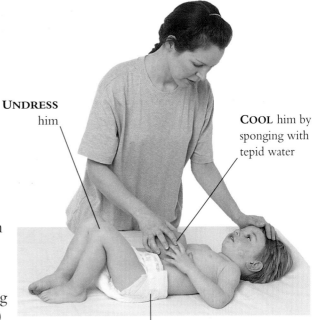

UNDRESS him

COOL him by sponging with tepid water

LET his skin dry in the air

> **FEVER** *can also be caused by too much sun; see* HEATSTROKE, *p.98.*

101

SPONGE her down

LET her skin dry in the air

Meningitis

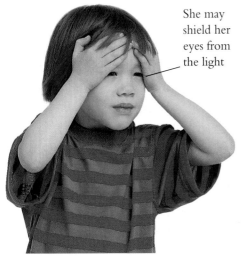

She may shield her eyes from the light

This is an inflammation of the tissues that surround the brain. It is a very serious condition and must be treated promptly.

Recognizing meningitis • *Fever* • *Listlessness* • *Vomiting* • *Loss of appetite* • *Headache or, in babies, a swollen "soft spot" at the top of the skull* • *Pain in eyes from light* • *Pain and stiffness in the neck* • *Convulsions* • *A rash of red or purple blood spots* • *A change for the worse in a child who has recently had an infection.*

Make your child comfortable, lying back against pillows or cushions.
☎ CALL 911 OR YOUR LOCAL EMS.

VOMITING

HOLD a bowl
for her

> **A BABY** *suffering repeated vomiting and*
> *diarrhea can become dangerously dehydrated.*
> *Prolonged vomiting may need to be treated with*
> *mineral replacement drinks.*
> ✚ TAKE YOUR BABY TO THE HOSPITAL

1 Hold your child over a bowl or basin.
Support her upper body with your free
hand while she vomits.
Reassure her.

SPONGE
her face
gently

2 Once she has
stopped vomiting,
wipe her face and
around her mouth
with a sponge or
cloth wrung out in
tepid water.

GIVE her fluid
to drink

3 Give her fluids to
replace any fluid loss and
to remove the unpleasant
taste. Encourage her to sip
each drink slowly.

LET her rest

4 Let her rest quietly, in
bed if she wants to.
Make sure the bowl is still
available for further vomiting
attacks, and provide a fresh
drink.

GIVE her
some fluids

LEAVE a bowl
for her

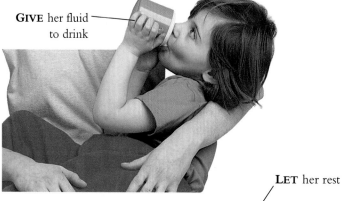

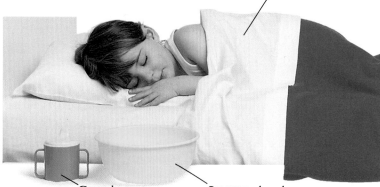

STOMACHACHE

PROP her up against cushions or pillows

1 Make your child comfortable on a sofa or bed. If she is having difficulty breathing, help her to lie back against cushions or pillows. She may want to vomit so leave a container nearby.

> **IF** *the pain is severe, or does not subside after 30 minutes, or if there are breathing problems,* ℂ CALL A DOCTOR.

PROVIDE a bowl in case she wants to vomit

GIVE her a covered hot-water bottle to hold against her stomach

2 Warmth may help relieve the pain. Fill a hot-water bottle – it must be covered – and give it to your child to hold against her stomach. Avoid giving her anything to eat.

103

Appendicitis

Inflammation of the appendix may affect children of any age.

Recognizing appendicitis • *Waves of pain in the middle of the abdomen* • *Acute pain settling in the right lower abdomen* • *Raised temperature* • *Loss of appetite* • *Nausea* • *Vomiting* • *Diarrhea.*

> **APPENDICITIS** *must be treated promptly. Help your child lie down on a sofa or bed. Do not give him anything to eat or drink.*
> ☎ CALL 911 OR YOUR LOCAL EMS

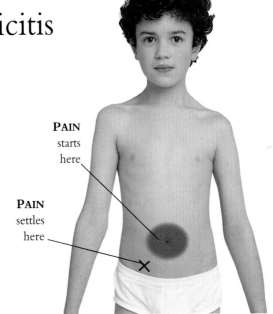

PAIN starts here

PAIN settles here

EARACHE

GIVE her recommended dose of liquid acetaminophen

1 Make your child comfortable. Sit her up supported by pillows or cushions if lying flat makes the earache worse. Give her the recommended dose of liquid acetaminophen.

PROP her up

2 Applying heat may help to soothe the pain. Prepare a covered hot-water bottle and tell your child to lie down with her painful ear against it.

IF *pain does not begin to subside, or if there is a discharge from the ear, fever, or a hearing loss,* ⓒ CALL A DOCTOR.

PROVIDE a covered hot-water bottle to hold against her ear

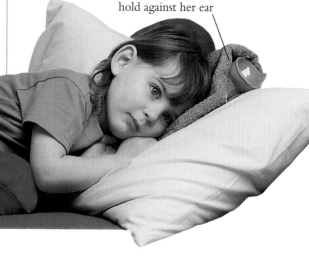

104

Pressure-change earache

This may happen on plane journeys, particularly when taking off or landing, or when traveling through tunnels. To make the ears "pop," your child should close her mouth, hold her nose, and blow. Sucking a piece of hard candy may also help. Allow babies to suck a bottle or pacifier.

TELL her to pinch her nose, close her mouth, and "blow" her nose

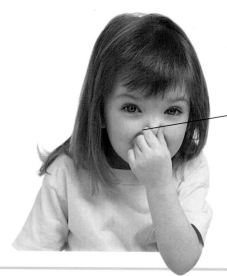

TOOTHACHE

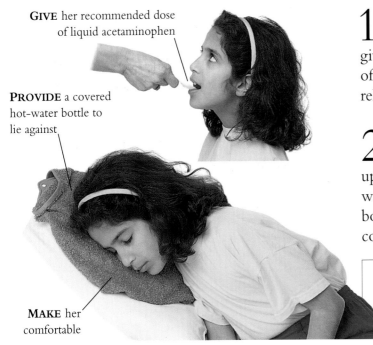

GIVE her recommended dose of liquid acetaminophen

PROVIDE a covered hot-water bottle to lie against

MAKE her comfortable

1 Arrange an appointment with your child's dentist. Meanwhile, give her the recommended dose of liquid acetaminophen to relieve the pain.

2 If lying down does not help to relieve the pain, prop your child up with pillows or cushions. The warmth of a covered hot-water bottle held against the cheek may comfort her.

IF *jaw is swollen and pain is severe,* Ⓒ CALL A DOCTOR.

CRAMP

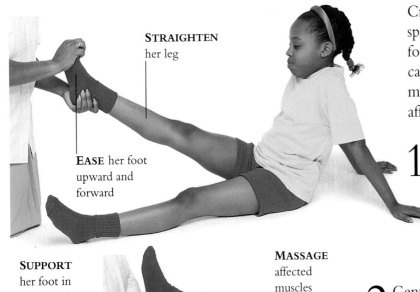

STRAIGHTEN her leg

EASE her foot upward and forward

SUPPORT her foot in your hand

MASSAGE affected muscles

Cramp is a painful muscle spasm that often affects the foot and calf muscles. You can relieve the pain by massaging and stretching the affected muscles.

1 Help your child to sit down, then raise her leg and straighten her knee. Ease her toes upward to flex the foot.

2 Gently but firmly massage the affected muscle with the palms of your hands until the spasm has passed completely.

FIRST AID KIT

A first aid kit
1 small roller bandage
1 large roller bandage
1 small conforming
  bandage
1 large conforming
  bandage
2 eye pads with
  bandages
Scissors
Calamine lotion
Pack of gauze swabs
2 triangular bandages
Hypoallergenic tape
2 sterile pads
*Waterproof adhesive
  bandages*
*1 finger bandage and
  applicator*
Tweezers
*1 sterile dressing with
  bandage*

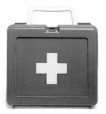

Keep first aid kits in your car and your home. You can buy a standard kit. You may want to add extra dressings and bandages, and disposable gloves. Make sure your first aid box is readily accessible and easy to identify, and check the contents regularly. Don't keep medicines in the first aid box; they should be locked in a medicine cabinet. A well-stocked kit might contain the articles shown below.

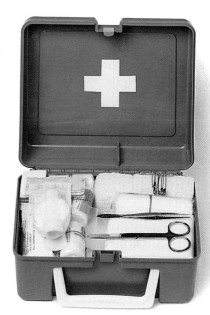

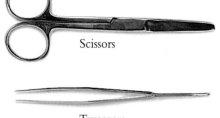

Scissors

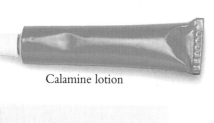

Tweezers

Dressings
Adhesive bandages are used for minor wounds. Keep several different sizes and shapes. Keep a selection of larger sterile dressings for more serious wounds.

Gauze swabs

Calamine lotion

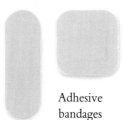

Adhesive
bandages

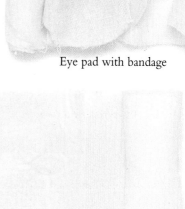

Eye pad with bandage

Sterile nonadhesive pad

Sterile dressing with bandage

Bandages

Keep a variety of bandages to secure dressings and support injured joints. Conforming bandages shape themselves to the contours of the body and so are easy to use. Triangular bandages can be used as slings and for binder and cravat bandages.

Hypoallergenic tape for securing dressings

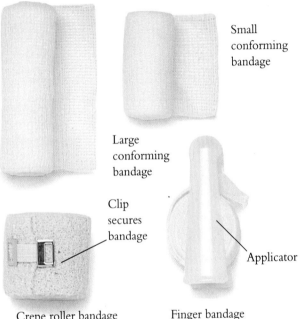

Small conforming bandage

Large conforming bandage

Clip secures bandage

Applicator

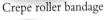

Crepe roller bandage

Finger bandage

Large roller bandage

Safety pins

Folded triangular bandage

Other useful items

A variety of household items are invaluable for first aid emergencies. If you don't have exactly the right materials, you can improvize successfully. Keep the following articles available.

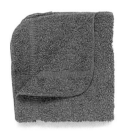

Washcloth
Use a washcloth soaked in water to make a cold compress or to sponge a child with a fever.

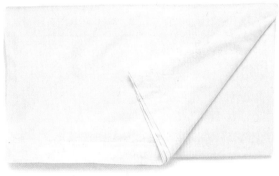

Sheet and pillowcase
A clean cotton sheet or pillowcase makes an excellent loose protective covering for burns.

Plastic wrap
This can be used to seal chest wounds.

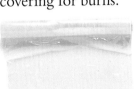

Plastic bags
A clean plastic bag can be put over a burned foot or hand and lightly secured with bandages or tape.

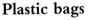

107

DRESSINGS

Adhesive bandage

Covering a wound with a dressing will help prevent infection and speed up the blood-clotting process. Dressings should not be fluffy and need to be large enough to cover the wound and the surrounding area. Always wash your hands before you apply dressings and wear disposable gloves if you have them. If blood soaks through a dressing, place another on top. Make sure any bandages are not too tight (see opposite).

Remove wrapping and, holding the pad over the wound, peel back the protective strips. Press the ends and edges down.

Sterile pad

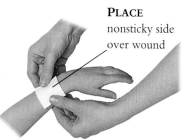

PLACE nonsticky side over wound

BANDAGE the pad in place

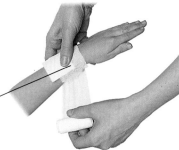

SECURE end of bandage with tape

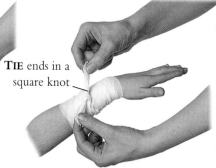

1 Place the pad shiny side down directly over the wound.

2 Secure the pad with a bandage, working from below the injury up the limb.

3 Secure the end of the bandage with hypoallergenic tape.

Sterile dressing with bandage

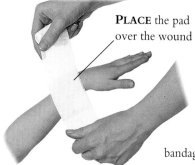

PLACE the pad over the wound

WIND the bandage up the limb

TIE ends in a square knot

1 Hold the bandage on each side of the dressing, and place the pad over the wound.

2 Leaving the short end hanging, wind the other end around the limb until the dressing is covered.

3 Tie the two ends of the bandage in a SQUARE KNOT (see p.76) over the pad.

BANDAGING

Use bandages to secure dressings, help control bleeding, and support injuries. Roller bandages can be used for any part of the body; conforming bandages are especially useful for bandaging joints or heads since they mold themselves to the shape of the body.

DO NOT *apply a bandage too tightly – it will impair the circulation. To check, press on your child's nail or a patch of skin beyond the bandage, then release pressure. The color should return rapidly; if not, loosen the bandages.*

Roller bandage

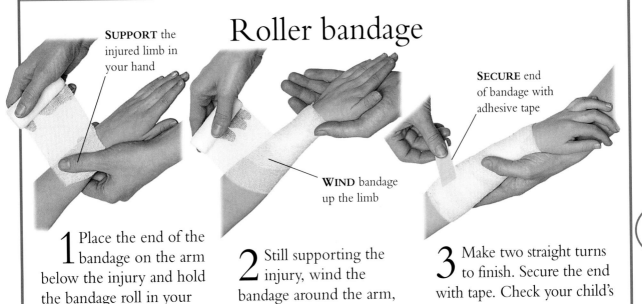

SUPPORT the injured limb in your hand

WIND bandage up the limb

SECURE end of bandage with adhesive tape

1 Place the end of the bandage on the arm below the injury and hold the bandage roll in your other hand.

2 Still supporting the injury, wind the bandage around the arm, winding up the limb.

3 Make two straight turns to finish. Secure the end with tape. Check your child's circulation (see above).

109

Hand bandage

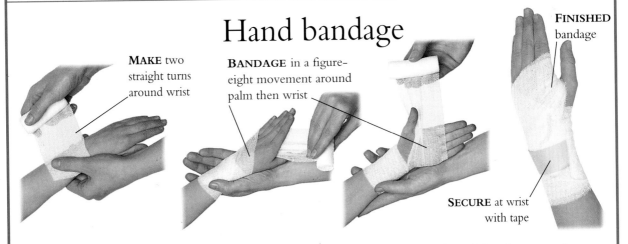

MAKE two straight turns around wrist

BANDAGE in a figure-eight movement around palm then wrist

FINISHED bandage

SECURE at wrist with tape

1 Supporting the injury, hold the end of the bandage on the wrist and make two straight turns.

2 Take the bandage across the back of the hand to the base of the little finger, then around the palm, and up between the thumb and forefinger, and across the back of the hand to the wrist. Repeat the figure-eight until the hand is covered.

TRIANGULAR BANDAGES

These are sold singly in sterile packs or can be made from a square of strong fabric folded diagonally in half. Triangular bandages are used for BINDER and CRAVAT BANDAGES (see p.76), or slings. Arm slings support injured arms or wrists, or take weight off an injured shoulder. Elevation slings can be used for arm and upper body injuries where bleeding, pain, or swelling need to be reduced. (For SQUARE KNOT see p.76.)

Arm sling

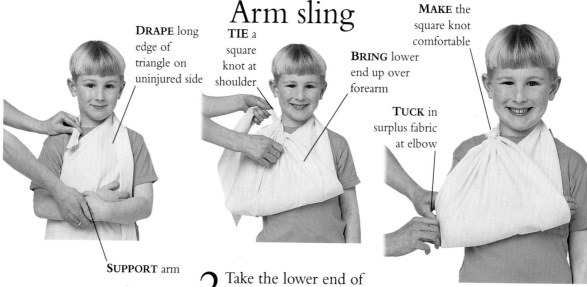

DRAPE long edge of triangle on uninjured side

SUPPORT arm

TIE a square knot at shoulder

BRING lower end up over forearm

MAKE the square knot comfortable

TUCK in surplus fabric at elbow

1 Place the bandage between your child's arm and chest, easing one end up around the back of his neck on the injured side.

2 Take the lower end of the bandage up over your child's forearm to the end at the shoulder and tie a SQUARE KNOT (see p.76) just below the shoulder.

3 Fold in the surplus fabric at the corner near the elbow and pin it to the bandage.

Improvised slings

If your child injures her shoulder, arm, or hand outdoors, you can improvise a sling to support the injury until she receives further treatment.

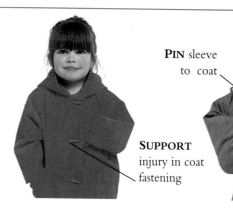

SUPPORT injury in coat fastening

PIN sleeve to coat

Undo a coat button and tuck the hand of the injured arm inside the fastening.

Alternatively, pin your child's sleeve up on the opposite side of his chest.

110

Elevation sling

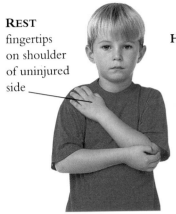

REST fingertips on shoulder of uninjured side

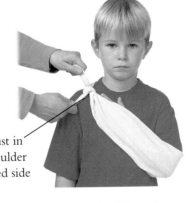

HOLD top corner at shoulder

DRAPE long edge across body

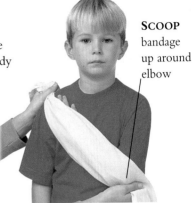

SCOOP bandage up around elbow

1 Have your child bring the arm on his injured side across his chest. Ask him to support his elbow.

2 Lay the bandage over your child's arm, with the long edge hanging on the uninjured side. Hold the top corner at the shoulder.

3 Fold long edge of bandage in under injured arm.

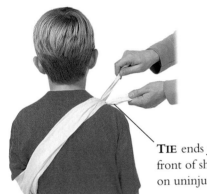

TIE ends just in front of shoulder on uninjured side

111

4 Bring the other end up around his back, holding the elbow securely in the fabric. Tie a SQUARE KNOT (p.76) just below the shoulder and tuck the ends in.

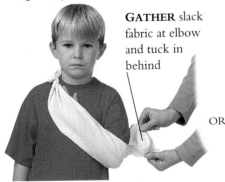

GATHER slack fabric at elbow and tuck in behind

OR

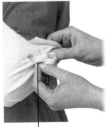

PIN slack fabric to front of sling

5 Secure the bandage by twisting the excess fabric and tucking it in at the elbow. Pin in place.

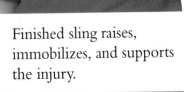

Finished sling raises, immobilizes, and supports the injury.

SAFETY IN THE HOME

Most accidents occur at home and over half involve children under the age of five. Many accidents are preventable if you:

- Alter the layout and position of objects and furniture at home.
- Make sure windows are closed or inaccessible, or have window guards.
- Never confuse containers by putting a dangerous substance, such as bleach, in a bottle that used to contain a harmless drink.
- Never tell your child that medicines and pills are special candies.
- Check for potential hazards when visiting friends or relatives and ask if you can move sharp or breakable objects.
- Teach your child basic safety rules.

ELECTRICITY

Protect your child from electric shock (see p.12):

- Cover sockets: put heavy furniture in front of them, or fit plastic covers.
- Put only one or two plugs into each socket – overloading can start a fire.
- Wire plugs safely – follow instructions and check that you have the right fuse.
- Check that old cords are not worn – a child may try to chew protuding wires.
- Coil trailing wires neatly.
- Fit a GFCI (ground fault circuit interrupter).

112

TEACH your child to recognize hazards

GAS

Find out where your gas valve is in case there is a leak. If you smell gas:

- Don't turn the lights on or off, or use any electric switches – there might be a spark that could cause an explosion.
- Don't light matches or cigarettes.
- Turn off the gas.
- Open the windows.
- Call the gas company and leave the house.

FIRE

If fire breaks out at home, it could be a matter of minutes before smoke overcomes you.

Install at least one smoke detector per floor If your house is on one level, fit a detector between the living room and the bedrooms. If your house is on two or more levels, fit one detector at the foot of the stairs and another outside the bedrooms upstairs.

Have an escape plan Make sure the whole family knows what to do if there is a fire. Teach older children to "stop, drop and roll" if their clothes catch fire (see p.11).

Practice a fire drill with your children
- Shout "fire" • Set off the smoke detector • Tell everyone to drop to the floor and crawl to the exit from the room • Shut the door behind you • Don't go back inside • Meet outside the house.

> **KEEP** *emergency numbers by the telephone, and make sure the babysitter knows where they are.*

HALL AND STAIRS

The staircase is not a safe place for your child to play (see below).
- Make sure that toys are not left there for you to trip over.
- Put a light in your hall or on the landing in case your child gets up at night. Use a low watt bulb, and never cover a lamp with a cloth since the cloth can easily catch fire.
- Don't let your child play on the landings or stairs of a communal area in apartment buildings, since the banisters may have large gaps between them.

FRONT DOOR
- Don't leave your front door open.
- Don't let your child open the door for strangers.
- Put the door knob out of reach of small children. If your toddler can reach the knob, fix an additional bolt higher up the door and always keep the door bolted.
- Glass doors should be made with toughened or laminated glass only.
- Put stickers on the glass to make it more noticeable for young children.

FLOOR
Tiled, polished, or sisal-covered floors can be very slippery for toddlers and running children.
- Put nonslip webbing under rugs.
- Keep hall floors free of toys and clutter.
- Check wall-to-wall carpets regularly for holes or loose areas that might catch a toddler's foot.

STAIRS
A child is not coordinated enough to be able to walk downstairs safely until he is at least three years old.
- Fit stair gates at the foot and top of the stairs. Vertical posts on stair gates should be no more than 2⅜in (6cm) apart. A young child can get through a larger gap and fall, or get his head stuck. Always open the gate when you are going upstairs or downstairs. Do not climb over it: your children will learn from you.
- Check your banisters for safety. Make sure the handrail is sturdy and check regularly for loose posts. Posts should be no more than 4in (10cm) apart. Do not let your child use the rails as a jungle gym.
- Check the stair carpet. Loose carpet or worn steps can be a hazard.

113

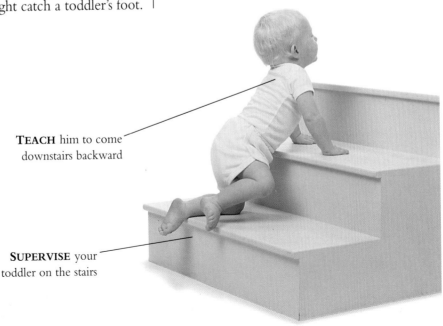

TEACH him to come downstairs backward

SUPERVISE your toddler on the stairs

KITCHEN

The kitchen may be the busiest part of your house, where you spend a lot of time with your children. Constant bustle and cooking activities make it a potentially hazardous area.

DOOR

- Any glass panels should be made of toughened or laminated glass in case your toddler runs into the door.
- Put some colorful stickers on the glass to alert your child.

FLOOR

- Don't let your child play on the area of floor between you and the work surface or where you could trip over him.
- Avoid bumps and falls by wiping up spills immediately.
- Remove pet food bowls after use and keep that part of the floor scrupulously clean.
- Clean up toys and clutter from underfoot.

TRASH CANS

- Discourage toddlers from rummaging in the garbage and trash cans.
- Put sharp-edged cans and lids or broken glass straight into the trash can.
- Keep the garbage can in a cabinet with a child-resistant safety catch.

> **KEEP** *a fire blanket in the kitchen for smothering flare-ups. If you want to buy a fire extinguisher, consult your local fire department to find out which is the most appropriate type. For more on fires, see p.11 and p.112.*

Babies

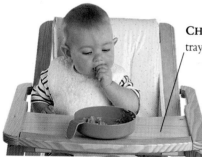

CHECK that removable trays have strong clasps

ATTACH a safety harness to the clips on either side of the chair

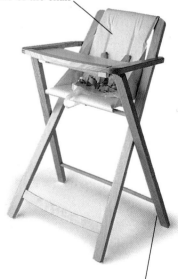

BOTTLES AND FOOD

- Sterilize all your baby's feeding equipment.
- Don't leave a prepared meal standing at room temperature, and don't keep the remains of the last feeding. Warmed or reheated meals are breeding grounds for bacteria that might upset your baby's stomach.

HIGHCHAIRS

- Always use a safety harness.
- Never leave the chair where your baby can reach out and pull objects down from a surface. Keep him amused with a safe toy.
- Never leave your child unattended.

PLAY

- Have a safe area or a playpen where your baby can play and watch you.
- Keep him out of range of any spills from the stove.

CHOOSE a stable highchair with widely spaced legs.

TABLES AND WORK SURFACES

- Always be aware of your child's reach and keep all heavy, breakable, or sharp objects well back from the edges of tables and work areas.
- Keep stools or chairs away from tables and work surfaces to prevent your child climbing up on them.
- Tuck cords of teapots, toasters, blenders, and irons out of reach. Choose a curly cord for your teapot if possible. It is not only boiling, steaming kettles that pose a hazard: water is still hot enough to scald 15 minutes after it has stopped boiling.
- Leave electrical appliances unplugged when they are not in use.
- Avoid using a tablecloth. It is tempting for a crawling baby or toddler to use it to pull himself up, bringing anything on the table down upon his head. Use place mats instead, or secure the cloth with clips.

CABINETS AND DRAWERS

- Put safety catches on cabinets and drawers, particularly those that contain: knives, scissors, and utensils; heavy pots, pans, or china; dried food, such as lentils or pasta, that may be a choking hazard; alcohol and bottles; medicines, including vitamins; cleaning materials, such as washing powder or bleach, including those with "child-resistant" lids.

REFRIGERATOR

Food poisoning can be caused by poor food storage. Take precautions to minimize risks:

- Keep cooked meat and poultry on a separate shelf from uncooked meat. Cover uncooked meat with plastic wrap.
- Don't store food in open cans; transfer leftovers into a clean container and put in the refrigerator.
- Check food regularly, to see that nothing is kept beyond the "sell by" date.

STOVE

Your child is obviously at risk of burns and scalds from hot fat or boiling water when you are preparing food.

- You can buy safety guards, but remember that a child can still poke fingers through them and be burned by hot electric or gas burners.
- Always keep your child away from oven doors; they can get very hot while the oven is in use and will stay hot for some time afterward. A crawling baby or toddler is particularly at risk. Try to teach your child what "hot" means, so that he understands a warning.
- Keep matches well out of reach in a cupboard with a safety catch.

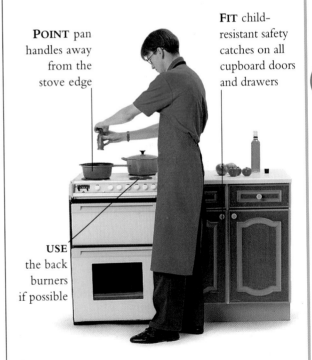

POINT pan handles away from the stove edge

FIT child-resistant safety catches on all cupboard doors and drawers

USE the back burners if possible

WASHING MACHINE AND TUMBLE DRIER

- Keep small hands away from the glass door; it may get hot while the machine is on.
- Ensure that the door is closed while the machine is not in use. Your toddler may try to climb inside, or fill it with toys.

115

LIVING ROOM

While your children are very young, try to arrange the room so that both children and your valuables are kept out of harm's way. If you have a balcony, block up gaps in the railings with particleboard and check that your child can't climb over. Never leave toys on a high surface since he may attempt to retrieve them.

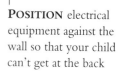

CARPETS AND CURTAINS

- Check that there are no areas of carpet or rug that have holes or turned up edges; either you or your child could trip.
- Wind up and tuck away curtain ties and cords for blinds. Children can be strangled if they get caught in dangling cords.

FIREPLACES AND HEATERS

- Don't leave matches or lighters where your child can reach them.
- Use a firescreen in front of an open fire. Fix it to the wall to prevent your child from pulling it over. Put a guard over gas heaters.
- Never use the firescreen as a shelf or clothes dryer.
- Use a spark-guard as well as a firescreen for open fires as an additional precaution.

TELEVISIONS, VIDEOS, AND STEREO EQUIPMENT

- Tack wiring to the baseboard.
- Run long cords behind furniture, so that your child won't trip or pull on them.
- Cover any unused plug sockets with plastic safety covers.
- Check that old cords are not worn.

POSITION electrical equipment against the wall so that your child can't get at the back

SURFACES AND FURNITURE

- Place houseplants out of reach of young children. Some houseplants are poisonous, and others can scratch or cause allergic reactions if touched.
- Keep breakable or heavy objects off low tables and well back from the edges of surfaces such as window sills or mantelpieces.
- Remove glass-topped tables and put corner protectors on sharp table corners.
- Don't leave hot drinks, alcohol, glasses, cigarettes, matches, or lighters on low surfaces, such as coffee tables, where your child can reach them.
- Keep alcohol in a locked cupboard.
- Never leave a cigarette burning on the arm of a sofa or armchair. Old foam furniture can be lethal in a fire since it releases toxic fumes within seconds of catching fire.

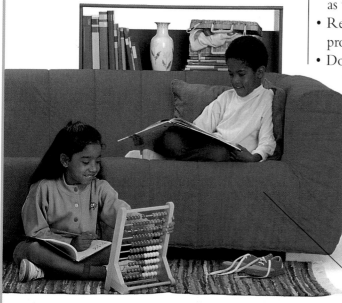

CHOOSE sofas and armchairs with fire-resistant upholstery and stuffing

TOYS AND PLAYTHINGS

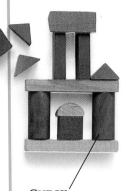

When you buy toys or equipment for your child, follow these guidelines:

- Buy toys that display the appropriate safety label and buy from a reputable source.
- Make sure that there are no sharp edges, and avoid anything made of thin, rigid plastic.
- Buy nontoxic paints or crayons.
- Don't buy your child second-hand toys: they may be covered in paint containing lead.
- Avoid novelty toys that are not designed for young children: look out for warnings on the packaging.

CHECK that sets of building blocks don't have small pieces that could be a choking hazard for your child

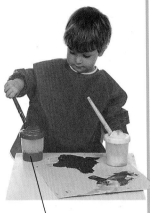

GIVE your child nontoxic paints and crayons

CARING FOR TOYS

- Check toys regularly and throw away any broken ones.
- Don't mix batteries – change them all at the same time; otherwise, the strong batteries will make the weak ones very hot.
- Keep toys in a toy box. Toys can cause accidents or injuries by being left on the floor.

117

Babies and toddlers

- Remove ribbons from a baby's soft toys.
- Check that the eyes, noses, ears, or bells on soft toys and dolls are well secured.
- Attach crib toys with a very short string.
- Remove activity centers or bulky toys from a crib as soon as your child can stand, since they provide a foothold for climbing out.
- Don't let babies chew on furry toys: the fur is a choking hazard for children under one year old.
- Never give a small child a toy that is not recommended for his age-group since it may contain small pieces on which he could choke.
- Always supervise a baby or toddler while he is playing.

MAKE SURE that toys that increase mobility are stable

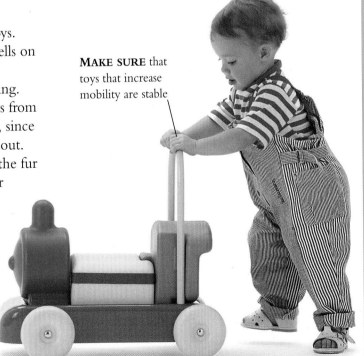

BEDROOMS

The closets and drawers in bedrooms are always exciting places for toddlers and young children. Make sure any potentially hazardous items are out of reach, because you may not always know when your child will decide to go exploring on his own.

Babies

CRIB

- Make sure the crib is deep enough to prevent your baby from climbing out – at least 1ft 8in (50cm) from the top of the mattress to the top of the crib.
- Bar spaces must be between 1–2½ in (2.5–6cm) wide to prevent your baby's head from being trapped.

- The mattress must be the right size with a gap no larger than 1½ in (3cm) around the side; otherwise, the baby's head could get trapped between the side of the crib and the mattress.
- Do not use a pillow for a baby under a year: it could suffocate him. If you need to raise his head, put a pillow underneath the mattress.
- Use a sheet and woven blankets, rather than a down comforter, until your baby is a year old. Your baby may get overheated or kick the comforter over his face and suffocate.
- Always put your baby to sleep on his back or side (never on his front) to lessen risk of crib death.
- Remove bumpers as soon as the baby can sit up – he could use them to climb out.
- Once he starts trying to climb out of the crib, transfer him to a bed. You can fit a bed guard at first, until he is used to the bed.

CHECK the crib dropside has strong clasps that your baby cannot open

ENSURE that bumpers have very short ties, to prevent strangulation

CHANGING AREA

- Keep all changing equipment in one area, so that you never have to leave your baby alone. He will be safest on the floor, but if you have a changing table, remember that he might roll off if left for even a moment.
- Do not have shelves above the changing area in case something falls off.
- Keep mobiles out of his reach.
- If you use talcum powder, sprinkle it on your hands and rub them together to avoid creating a cloud of dust around your baby.

CHANGE your baby on a changing mat on the floor so that he cannot fall

Your child's room

BEDS

- Use a bed guard when your toddler first moves to a bed.
- Top bunk beds must have safety rails on both sides and any gaps in the railings or between the top of the mattress and the bottom of the safety rail should be less than 3in (7.5cm).
- A top bunk is not recommended for children under the age of six.
- Never let young children play on the top bunk.
- Pick up toys from the floor around the bed at night.

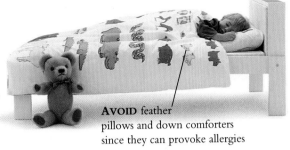

AVOID feather pillows and down comforters since they can provoke allergies

WINDOWS

Make sure your child can't climb out. Even if his room is on the ground floor, he is in danger if he falls.

- Attach a safety catch, but make sure the window can be opened easily in the event of a fire.
- Try not to place a piece of furniture under a window – it may encourage your child to climb up.

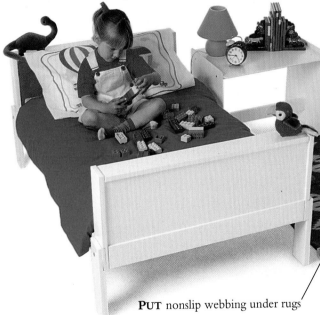

TOYS (see p.117).

- Try to keep toys with small pieces separate from others, so that you can easily remove them and put them out of reach for a while if your child is sharing a room with a toddler, or if you have young visitors.

PUT nonslip webbing under rugs

119

Your room

- **Medicines and pills** Do not keep them beside your bed or on a dressing table. Put them out of sight and out of reach.
- **Scissors and sewing equipment** Keep these in a drawer or cupboard where your child cannot reach them.
- **Perfume, hairspray, and makeup** These can be harmful if sprayed or rubbed in the eyes, or drunk, so keep them out of reach, or in a drawer with a safety catch.
- **China cups and glasses** Never leave a china cup or a glass on the floor by your bed. If your child is sleeping in your bed at night and rolls out onto the cup or the glass, he could have a serious accident.

BATHROOMS

Your child may be at risk from falls, drowning, or poisoning in the bathroom. Keep the bathroom door shut at all times to discourage him from going in. On the inside of the door, attach the bolt high up, to prevent a small child from locking himself in.

SHOWER
- Keep a constant check on the temperature of the water.
- Use nonslip mats in the shower and on the bathroom floor.
- Glass shower doors should be made of toughened or laminated glass.

BATH
- Always check the temperature of the water before your child gets in. A young child can be badly scalded by hot bathwater.
- Use nonslip mats in the bath and on the floor by the bath.
- Never leave a young child or baby alone in the bath. A baby can drown in just 1in (2.5cm) of water. If you need to answer the doorbell or telephone, take your child with you.

CABINETS
- Store bathroom chemicals and other potential poisons, such as toilet cleaners and bleach, out of reach in a cabinet with a safety catch.
- Keep other hazards, such as makeup, aftershave, razors, nail scissors, and any medicines or glass containers, out of reach in a locked medicine cabinet.

TOILET
- Use a special child toilet seat adaptor and step for toddlers, so that they can keep their balance more easily and so feel more secure.
- Keep the toilet seat closed.
- Don't use block toilet cleaners that a small child could pull out and chew.
- Never mix toilet cleaners with bleach since this can give off toxic fumes.
- If your toddler uses a potty, keep it clean, but never leave bleach or cleaning agents inside it.

BATH him away from the tap end

NEVER leave your child unattended in the bath

USE a nonslip mat in the bath

GARDEN

You don't have to be an enthusiastic gardener to make your garden into a safe and interesting place for children to play. Children will find their own corners to play in but you should remove obvious hazards:

- Clear away any trash or rubble.

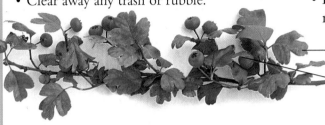

- Check garden furniture or play equipment regularly to make sure that it is stable and safe.
- Keep pets out of areas where children play.
- Make sure paving is even and remove moss on which children may easily trip or slip.
- Lock gates that lead out of the garden and make sure fences are secure.

WARN your child never to eat berries or leaves

PLANTS

Many plants are poisonous if eaten and digested in large quantities. Small pieces, or one or two berries, may not be fatal, but may cause some discomfort and stomach upset.

- Tell your child about the dangers of eating berries and keep babies and toddlers away from them.
- Remove plants that you know to be poisonous, such as deadly nightshade, laburnum, and toadstools.
- Cut back any prickly plants, such as roses, brambles, and holly – they can give nasty scratches, especially to the eyes.

SUPERVISE your toddler at all times. Check that he is playing in a clean, safe area with safe toys

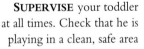

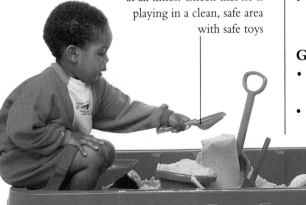

SHEDS

These are exciting dens for children.

- If your shed is full of gardening equipment or tools, tell your child that it is out of bounds and keep it locked.
- Put any chemicals, such as weedkiller or slug pellets and insecticides, out of reach.

PONDS, WADING POOLS, AND WATER BARRELS

Children are in danger if they slip and fall, even in shallow water.

- Never leave children unattended when they are playing in, or near, water.
- Cover ponds, water barrels, and empty trash cans that collect rainwater.
- Always empty out a wading pool when the children have finished playing in it.

GARDENING

- Don't apply chemicals when children will be playing in the garden.
- Don't mow the lawn while children are close by, since stone chips may be dislodged and fly into their eyes.
- Fit circuit breakers on all electrical equipment such as mowers and hedgetrimmers.
- Put away all garden tools when you have finished using them.

OUT AND ABOUT

After the home, most accidents to children occur on the street. Teach your child the rules of the road from an early age, reminding him to stay alert for traffic and to cross in a safe place. It takes a long time for children to develop a true road sense.

BY THE ROAD

- Three-year-olds can learn that sidewalks are safe and the road is dangerous.
- Five-year-olds can learn how to cross the road, but they are still not able to put this knowledge into practice on their own.
- Eight-year-olds can cross quiet streets on their own, but are not yet able to judge the speed and distance of traffic.
- Twelve-year-olds can judge the speed of an oncoming car, but are still easily distracted by friends.

IN THE STREET

Whenever you are out with your child, show him how to be aware of his own safety.

- Use reins or a wrist strap for a toddler, to keep him from running off.
- Hold a child's hand when you are near the road, or waiting to cross.
- Teach your child by your example and always find a safe place to cross. This may be:

  ▲ *A zebra crossing – wait at the island midway, if there is one.*

  ▲ *A traffic light. Encourage your child to press the button, if there is one, and tell him to wait until the traffic has stopped.*

  ▲ *An underpass.*

  ▲ *A footbridge or overpass.*

  ▲ *A corner at an intersection.*

Crossing the road

Teach your child the rules of the road.

▲ *Find a safe place to cross, then stop.*

▲ *Stand on the pavement, near the curb.*

▲ *Look all around for traffic, and listen.*

▲ *If traffic is coming, let it pass.*

▲ *When there is no traffic near, walk straight across the road.*

▲ *Keep looking and listening for traffic while you cross.*

BIKES

- Children younger than 11 years old should not bicycle on roads in traffic.
- Arrange for your child to have bicycle training before he rides on the roads.
- Make sure your child can be seen when he's riding his bike – with bright fluorescent colors by day and reflectors on his clothes and bike by night. He should have an approved helmet to protect his head.

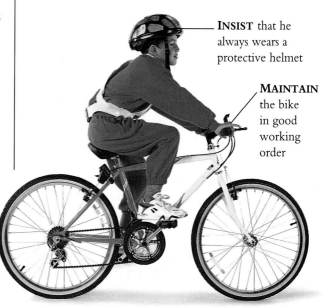

INSIST that he always wears a protective helmet

MAINTAIN the bike in good working order

122

PLAYING

What may seem common sense to you, is not always obvious to children.

- Teach your child the dangers of playing in open areas such as roads, building sites, and quarries.
- Tell your child not to play in the street, or on a sidewalk near the curb.
- Tell him that he must never chase a ball, a pet, or another child into the road.
- Tell him not to try to cross the road from between two closely parked cars.

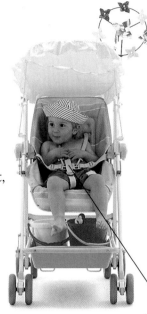

HARNESS your baby into his stroller

STROLLERS AND CARRIAGES

- Never push a stroller or carriage out into the traffic – pull it to one side and check whether it is safe to cross. Remember that a carriage sticks out in front of you at least 3ft (1m).
- When you park a stroller or carriage, put on the brakes and point it away from traffic.
- Never tie your dog to the stroller.
- Never leave a baby unattended.

In the playground

Playgrounds should comply with safety standards and recommendations.

- The play area must be safely fenced off, away from roads.
- There should be a soft, even surface, such as bark chips or rubber tiles around equipment.
- Slides should be no higher than 8ft (2.4m) and preferably constructed on an earth mound to break any falls.
- Merry-go-rounds should be low, with a smooth surface, designed so that children can't get their feet stuck underneath.
- Jungle gyms or bars should be no higher than 8ft (2.4m), be completely stable and built over sand or a very soft surface to break falls.
- There should be a clearly defined area for toddlers and young children, set away from the more boisterous activities of older children.
- There should be someone to contact if equipment is faulty.
- Dogs must not be allowed inside.
- Make sure that children are always supervised by a responsible adult.

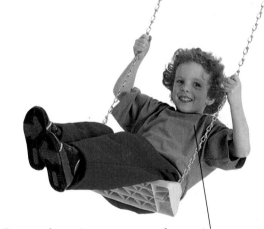

CHECK that swings are set apart from main play equipment, or fenced off, to prevent children running in front of, or behind, them

MAKE SURE your child is wearing suitable clothing

TEACH your child how to use equipment properly

STRANGERS *Remind your child of the dangers of talking to strangers. Have a code word that a friend can use if meeting your child. Tell your child not to go with anybody unless they use the code.*

GARAGE & CAR SAFETY

GARAGE

- Keep the garage locked and discourage your child from going in there.
- Keep equipment, chemicals, or tools out of your child's reach and locked away, if possible.
- Make sure you know where your child is when you are driving into, or out of, the garage.
- If you keep a freezer in the garage, it should be locked at all times.

CAR

- Never leave a young child unattended in a car.
- Don't let your child play with the window, whether manual or electric. Electric windows can trap a child's head or fingers.
- Remove the cigarette lighter.
- Watch out for your child's fingers when you shut the doors.
- Use child locks on rear doors until your child is at least six years old.
- Teach your child to get out of the car on the curb side.
- If your child is helping you as you wash or clean up the car, make sure you have removed the keys from the ignition.

CAR SEATS

Always put your child into a special safety seat when you strap him into the car. If you are buying a second-hand car seat, you must buy one that has a known history. Some car seats are reconditioned after a crash and will not be safe. Choose the right seat for the age of your child.

- **Babies** up to 22lb (10kg) – about nine months – should travel in a rear-facing car seat. The baby is harnessed into the seat and the seat is held in place by the car seatbelts. You can put this seat on the front passenger seat unless there is a passenger-side airbag. Your baby will be able to see you as you drive and is less likely to become upset from loss of contact with you.
- Never carry a baby on your lap, or inside your own seatbelt: he would be crushed in a crash.
- **Older babies and toddlers**, up to 40lb (18kg), need a molded car seat in the back. Some of these seats have an integral harness for the child that fits over his shoulders and between his legs. These seats are kept in place by the adult seat belt, or by straps that you can fasten into the car. Other seats use the adult belt to hold both child and seat into the car.
- **Primary school children** (from four or five years old up to about 11 years old) should travel in a booster seat. Without it, adult seat belts are neither comfortable nor safe. The shoulder part cuts across the child's neck and the lap strap lies across his stomach. In a crash, the lap strap can damage his liver or spleen. A booster seat raises a young child so the shoulder part lies across his upper chest and the lap strap lies across his hips. A lap strap on its own is not sufficient as it does not restrain the child's upper body.

FIT a molded car seat for maximum protection

INDEX

127

Acknowledgments

**British Red Cross
First Aid Training Department:**
Mr. Anthony Kemp, Miss Lyn Covey
Mr. Joe Mulligan

Safety in the home: advice on content, and text read by Dr. Sara Levene of the Child Accident Prevention Trust

Dorling Kindersley would like to thank:

Lorna Damms and Ros Fishel for editorial help; Sarah Ashun and Gary Ombler for assisting the photographers; Wendy Holmes for makeup; Hilary Bird for the index; the following for modeling:

Children Aleena Awan (4), Navaz Awan (3), Amy Davies (9), Thomas Davies (7), James Dow (6), Kyla Edwards (6), Austin Enil (5), Lia Foa (11), Maya Foa (9), Kashi Gorton (7), Emily Gorton (4), Thomas Greene (5), Alexander Harrison (7), Rupert Harrison (5), Ben Harrison (2), Jessica Harris-Voss (3), Jake Hutton (3 months), Rosemary Kaloki (10), Winnie Kaloki (8), Ella Kaye (11), Maddy Kaye (9), Jade Lamb (3), Emily Leney (5), Harriet Lord (3), Ailsa McCaughrean (4), Fiona Maine (9), Tom Maine (6), Maija Marsh (4), Oliver Metcalf (4), Eloise Morgan (3), Tom Razazan (9), Jimmy Razazan (7), Rebecca Sharples (8), Ben Sharples (6), Thomas Sharples (4), Ben Walker (10), Robyn Walker (8), Amy Beth Walton Evans (2), Hanna Warren-Green (5), Simon Weekes (6), Joseph Weir (2)

Adults Shaila Awan, Georgina Davies, Marion Davies, Sophie Dow, Tina Edwards, Rachel Fitchett, Emma Foa, Caroline Greene, Claire le Bas, Susan Harrison, Victoria Harrison, Julia Harris-Voss, Emma Hutton, Helga Lien Evans, Sylvie Jordan, Jane Kaloki, David Kaye, Louise Kaye, Geraldine McCaughrean, Diana Maine, Brian Marsh, Jonathon Metcalf, Francoise Morgan, Hossein Razazan, Angela Sharples, John Sharples, Vanessa Walker, Catherine Warren-Green, Toni Weekes.

Make-up: Pebbles, Geoff Portas

Additional photographs
Dave King, Ray Mollers, Suzannah Price, Dave Rudkin, Steve Shott

EMERGENCY TELEPHONE NUMBERS

IN AN EMERGENCY DIAL 911 OR YOUR LOCAL EMERGENCY NUMBER. ASK FOR THE POLICE, AMBULANCE, OR FIRE DEPARTMENT

DOCTOR
Name: _____
Address: _____

Telephone: _____
Office Hours: _____

POISON CONTROL CENTER
Center Address: _____

Telephone: _____
Center Hours: _____

HOSPITAL EMERGENCY DEPARTMENT
Address: _____

Telephone: _____

DENTIST
Name: _____
Address: _____

Telephone: _____
Office Hours: _____

EMERGENCY MEDICAL SERVICE (EMS)
Telephone: _____

LATE NIGHT PHARMACY
Address: _____

Telephone: _____

LOCAL POLICE STATION
Address: _____

Telephone: _____

GAS EMERGENCY SERVICE
Telephone: _____

ELECTRICITY EMERGENCY SERVICE
Telephone: _____

WATER EMERGENCY SERVICE
Telephone: _____

IN CASE OF AN EMERGENCY PLEASE CALL: _____

American Red Cross

The American Red Cross runs first aid and CPR courses for all ages.
For further information, get in touch with your local chapter;
you will find the number in the telephone directory.

128